On Blossoming

On Blossoming

Frank and Practical Advice on Our Bodies, Sexual Health, Sensuality, Pleasure, Orgasm, and More

Gia Lynne

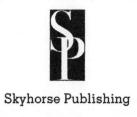

Skyhorse Publishing

Skyhorse Publishing books may be purchased in bulk at special discounts for sales promotion, corporate gifts, fund-raising, or educational purposes. Special editions can also be created to specifications. For details, contact the Special Sales Department, Skyhorse Publishing, 307 West 36th Street, 11th Floor, New York, NY 10018 or info@skyhorsepublishing.com.

Skyhorse® and Skyhorse Publishing® are registered trademarks of Skyhorse Publishing, Inc.®, a Delaware corporation.

Visit our website at www.skyhorsepublishing.com.

10 9 8 7 6 5 4 3 2 1

Library of Congress Cataloging-in-Publication Data is available on file.

Cover design by Daniel Brount

Print ISBN: 978-1-5107-4491-2
Ebook ISBN: 978-1-5107-4493-6

Printed in the United States of America

This book is dedicated to everyone who wants more.

CONTENTS

DISCLAIMER

My intent in writing this book is to change the conversation around sexuality to one that incorporates the principles of pleasure into sex education for youth. This book details my personal experiences with and viewpoints about human sexuality. I aim for you to find information, ideas, and tools that are useful to make healthy, responsible choices and add your voice to this significant conversation.

As you consider the information I offer and how it applies to your life, please remember that no book can replace parental guidance or professional counselling, education, health, and mental care. It is extremely important to consult with your own doctor before making any medical decisions. I and my publisher specifically disclaim any liability in connection with the use or application of the information in this book.

I have done my best to provide complete and accurate references in this book as of press time, including URLs, but of course websites do change over time.

• • • • • •

This is a work of creative nonfiction. While all the stories in this book are true, some names and identifying details have been changed to protect the privacy of the people involved.

Introduction

MY FUNDAMENTALS

Who here actually learned about pleasure when they were growing up? For that matter, who learned about their clitoris?" Andrea Barrica, founder of the online sex education platform O.school, looked across the packed room of educators, researchers, and sex ed enthusiasts who were attending her class on "Queering up Sex Ed." Sitting in the front row, I raised my hand, alone in doing so amongst roughly forty or so adults. She scanned the crowd, a smile already playing across her face, fully expecting to see no raised hands, and upon finding me, paused only momentarily to dismiss what she saw with a laughing quip, "There's always one, and they're always from the Netherlands!"

She's not entirely wrong, despite the fact that the majority of parents[1] would like their children to receive comprehensive sex education, and researchers have concluded that learning about pleasure is an integral aspect of sex education and healthy adulthood.[2] Yet, most people growing up and educated in the United States *do not* learn about pleasure at all.[3] In fact, most are fortunate to receive any kind of sex education, as only thirteen US states require sex education to be medically accurate and half of our youth do not even learn about contraception before they begin having sex.[4]

But she was wrong about the Netherlands thing. I was born and raised in Northern California by an intelligent group of individuals who believe in all people learning about their bodies and their personal potential for pleasure. Needless to say, I had a far more comprehensive sex education than many. I had one-on-one conversations with both of my parents about how bodies work, an actual homeschool class (comprised of my sister and I as the entire student body) called "The Female Body Class" where we learned about, you guessed it, all matters concerning our bodies, and was encouraged through conversation, my parents' actions, and the very environment I was immersed in to simply be myself, be a free person, and to love my own body.

• • • • • •

As an adult, I recognize the growing desire for a bigger, more inclusive conversation about pleasure with our youth. A disparity exists in our education: For the most part, girls learn about painful periods and unwanted pregnancies while boys learn about wet dreams and ejaculation, which results in an even greater disparity in adulthood. This occurs inside and outside of the bedroom: 95 percent of heterosexual men experience orgasm during most of their sexual encounters whereas heterosexual women experience orgasm 65 percent of the time,[5] yet, this disparity is even more apparent in larger social outcomes: youth (ages twelve to thirty-four) are at the highest risk of any age group to experience sexual assault, and one in six women will be the victim of rape or attempted rape within her lifetime.[6] It is my firm belief that comprehensive sex education focused on pleasure, which includes topics like body awareness, body image, pleasurable anatomy, positive communication skills, and tools to explore one's own body, is the key to changing the current taboo climate around our sexuality and sensuality. Learning about pleasure openly and encouraging positive, healthy choices in our early education creates more positive experiences and promotes sexual health in our adulthood and throughout our lives.

• • • • • •

When I was eight years old, I conceived of the idea of writing a book. As in, I realized that a person could actually write a book, a *whole book*. It seemed to be an enormous feat and an accomplishment worth doing in one's life. At around the same time, I wrapped my head around the concept of going to college for four years, which seemed like an interminable amount of time, and decided that was also a worthwhile endeavor. At age eight, I had two life goals set for myself.

I knew then that I lived a life to tell about: I was surrounded by happy adults living in community and I already knew that we had something fun going on. This seemed like a book that should be written.

Around that time, my dad taught me how to use our handheld camcorder. That night, as we sat around the barbecue fire lit only by the glowing coals, he told me that it is important for me to document. I didn't fully comprehend what he meant at the time (document what, exactly?) but I knew enough to listen and to follow his words. I stood there, holding the small camcorder in slightly shaky hands, and I watched a conversation unfold between adults, between friends. Their words didn't pertain to me, but I could stand back and observe, regardless of content. That notion of documentation, of acknowledging our experience together, has stuck with me ever since.

I realized when I got older that not everyone grew up the way I did. It was easy to see simply in what people knew about sex that I grew up knowing a lot more about how bodies work and how humans relate than was the norm. I realized that a lot of people my age didn't necessarily have good relationships with their parents even in their twenties, let alone through their teens. And that was perfectly fine, a sore spot perhaps, but nothing for them to change. I realized that most people don't want to talk about sex, *good sex*, despite the fact that they may be willing to joke about it or watch it online in the form of pornography. It seemed that there was a disconnect between how people thought of their bodies and how they experienced them.

In contrast, I grew up being friends with my parents. I was able to talk to both my mom and my dad about my body, about how I felt, and about what I noticed in the world around me. They taught me how to do that through telling me the truth about their own experience—what they thought, what they felt, what they were experiencing, what they were noticing.

Of course, they didn't tell me everything. At times I'd ask questions that I knew they wouldn't answer (like—what were you doing in your bedroom?) and my dad would reply, "I'll tell you when you're older." That was a rare occasion though, because he wanted my sister and I to know everything. How the world works, how people work, how our bodies work. He filled us with as much information as we'd possibly accept so that we could enter the world fully capable.

So, when I realized how differently most people were raised from the way I was, I thought I could do some good by writing about my experience and peppering in some need-to-know basics like (spoiler alert) how to masturbate and how to have safe sex.

My sister and I started this book when we were simultaneously in the throes of puberty ourselves: I was thirteen and she was fourteen. Our friend—also one of our homeschool teachers—moderated the project by giving us specific writing prompts around our book idea and designating amounts of time in which to write. It was a fascinating experience to answer questions that I was in the midst of exploring myself. She asked us questions about sex, the senses, our experience of our bodies changing, and our viewpoints on friendship. The content of our essays, while not grammatically correct or particularly eloquent, was raw and based entirely on feeling. I have not used any of that material directly, but the intention behind the original draft certainly made its way into this version.

My parents and their friends started the intentional community that I grew up in about ten years before I was born. An *intentional community* in this instance means a group of people who have deliberately decided to live together and share a common philosophy and have common goals. As our community formed, some of the founding members took courses from another successful community and teaching group. This is where they got a lot of the foundational information from which our community started. We took aspects of their information and ran with it in our own way, particularly around researching sensuality and friendship. The initial founding members got a ball rolling that has kept moving since then—people have moved in and out of our group, thousands of people from all over the world have come to study with us, and many, many lives have been changed. My Mom moved in during the eighties and eventually I came along. This is all to say that I come from a long line of people dedicated to fun and pleasurable living.

I'm not here to promote my community, but it is intricately intertwined with who I am. I have spent my whole life telling the truth, being told the truth, and talking openly about sex and sensuality—it's formed who I am today. Some of the founding members of my community formed a teaching group called "The Welcomed Consensus"; they are highly trained individuals who teach and research the viewpoints that I was brought up with and which I describe in this book. Dedicated to leading fun lives and doing it through "consensus," or, agreement, these people spend a lot of time talking, let me tell you. Hours are spent meeting together, discussing their lives and the lives of people in our community. They tell each other the truth about everything, which they use as a tool to create a sense of closeness and to improve their lives together. Telling the truth is simply the most efficient way to function and it's also the most fun.

My dad told me once that he had seen many smart, successful people in life that were not happy. We've had a full spectrum of people come through our community: home-makers and lawyers, authors and airline pilots, and entrepreneurs. Many have been the kind of people that followed the rules and did everything "right" by our society's standards: they got a steady job, found a good partner, had a couple of kids. But, still, they were unhappy. My dad taught me early on that regardless of how well-educated a person is, or how wealthy or worldly they are, it does not really matter unless they have figured out how to be happy. The rest of it, the degrees and the promotions, have nothing to do with happiness. My parents showed me each day how to be happy and how to lead a life that keeps getting better.

When I grew up, I realized that not all little girls are told about my favorite M's: masturbation and menstruation. We do not have enough positive voices about sexuality, let alone *female* sexuality. Porn and high school sex ed aren't enough. We must be given information and the tools necessary to truly enjoy our lives and our sexuality to the fullest potential.

One of the most important differences between the rest of the population, including other sex educators, and me, is that I am oriented toward fun. My dad told me when I was a kid that fun is an honorable goal. As a six-year-old, that made complete sense. My whole life was about fun anyways: from swimming in the creek to going to homeschool in our little one room schoolhouse in the backyard to sitting in on the house meetings that all my favorite adults would put on every few days. I think a lot of kids experience life this way: things are taken care of for you mostly and you're left to do the fun stuff. But when you start becoming an adult, you're told that you must face facts and grow up. We're told this in a myriad of ways, some more covertly than others.

My grandma was visiting one day, and, during her stay with us, she pulled me aside to tell me that I wouldn't always be climbing trees and wrestling with my cousin. She assured me that one day, I would not be so wild. I looked at her like she was crazy. I stood there, tiny in my pre-pubescence, thick, wild hair filled with sticks and whatever else the woods left me, and certainly shirtless because that was my daily preference at the time. I had just crawled out of the apple tree that grew in our front yard and my skin was itchy from rolling around on the grass earlier. She looked down at me and told me I would surely change. And when she said it, I concluded that this had something to do with getting a period. I didn't have one yet, but I figured the change she was going on about had something to do with that. I didn't truly comprehend what she was telling me at the time; all I knew was that I disagreed.

And, ultimately, I was right. I still climb trees and run around naked. But I don't think it goes like that for most women. When you're a girl, it's okay to be messy and loud and chubby. There's even a somewhat-dated term for girls that want to be wild: "tomboy." But once you begin showing signs of womanhood, you've got to straighten up. We're taught to be kind. We must be neat. We must be tidy. We must not talk too much or be too loud. And that's just no fun.

We are not taught how to be fun or how to have fun in our culture. Certainly, having fun as a goal seems quite frivolous and downright flakey from the collective societal viewpoint, especially after childhood and adolescence. "Fun" seems to be about having the latest iPhone or whatever gadget is the greatest. That's not what fun is, just like getting the right job doesn't guarantee your happiness. Nor are we taught how to be real friends and how to build friendships that last a lifetime and keep getting better.

My mom went into labor at my sister's first birthday party. There are a few pictures from the day; my sister's sparse, curly hair lightly decorating her big, round head, her body encased in a frilly white dress, and her big brown eyes looking straight into the camera. Her cousins and a few other babies were also in attendance. You can see them sprawled out on the rug or stuffing their greasy, food-filled hands into open mouths. I love these pictures in part because I know there is a story about to unfold: they mark the last day Sophia and I would be apart. We grew up together, more together than most, I'd say. We've shared a room our whole lives, we were homeschooled together at the same oversized desk, we even took college classes together and got the same degree. More than just the time spent together is the way that I feel for her—she is an integral part of me. Our parents did me an enormous favor by giving me a best friend right from the beginning.

This book is in essence an exploration of the tools for happiness, fun, and friendship, disguised as a sex ed book for young people. This book is part how-to and part how-I-did-it, a mix of memoir and straightforward information on the mechanics of sex and how to have successful relationships with people that can keep getting better over time. In order to lead a happy, sensually fulfilling life, it's critical to know how your body functions from a pleasure-oriented perspective. And I think that the more you know about your body, the better choices you'll make when it comes to the sensual experiences that you decide to have.

When people hear how I grew up, they often ask me how to talk to their teen about sex ed, or what I think the main messages in that realm should be for young people. My first reaction is usually to balk slightly, because those are huge, gigantic questions that, by virtue of being asked in short sentences, suggest that there could be a tidy, elevator-pitch-length response. And if that's why you picked up this book, then I hate to disappoint you, but that's impossible for two main reasons.

The first is that there is no "One-Size-Fits-All" to sex education; like knit caps on a store's clothing rack, we can't all simply choose our color and walk away happy. That's just not realistic. Everyone is different: we have different genders and different forms of sexual expression, we come from different areas of the world and different cultures, and we have a range of ages and ranges in experience. What I can offer, and what I explore in this book, is a perspective on pleasure that I know works and I have yet to see represented in our mainstream culture.

The second part is that my views on sexuality aren't for everyone. I decided to write my perspective on human sensuality and sexuality because it's different:

as I've mentioned, I was raised by a community of adults who taught courses on sensuality and communication, for starters. But I also had an excellent adolescence overall, which took me until my late twenties to fully appreciate. So, I decided that writing from the perspective of personal success would be something of value. I have done my best to describe my story because I think it's useful: we must change the collective conversation we have about pleasure in order to create positive change in the world. My view is that if we learn to value pleasure early on in our lives, there will be a positive impact on our shared experience and on our global community.

One of the central aims of my book is to answer the question "what comes after consent?" raised by Peggy Orenstein in her important book, *Girls & Sex*.[7] I plan to answer this question by describing *what comes before it*. Before we get into a position of saying "yes" or "no" to sex, or asking for sex, there is much to learn. Knowing about our bodies, knowing what pleasures us, and knowing how to communicate about these aspects improves all areas of our life.

And for the parents, guardians, and the shapers of youth reading this, let me say that *you* are one of the biggest teaching tools, so way to go for picking this up! As humans, we learn from each other. We're constantly watching one another and making choices based on what we see. If you are informed about sensuality and hold pleasure-based views yourself, it will have a positive effect on not just your own life, but also on the people around you.

So, while I do not aim to offer a comprehensive map of all-things sex education, what I can offer is the start of an ongoing conversation between you and the people you care about. Sex ed isn't a class, it's not a book, it's not a website: it's a *conversation*. It's a subject to relate over with your friends, guardians, lovers, peers, or with whomever you feel comfortable speaking. It's a conversation because we're constantly changing: our views, our experiences, and the choices we make all affect how we view our own sexuality. As we grow and have more life experiences, our view of sexuality morphs right along with us. So, what I aim to do with this book is to build a strong foundation of information for our youth of today and tomorrow to jump-start this conversation because it's truly a lifelong pursuit.

On Blossoming

Chapter 1
SENSUALITY AND SEXUALITY

Growing up, I was taught how important it was to deliberately choose what language I was going to use. My dad demonstrated through his own use of language and in the way he spoke with me that this was an area to pay attention to myself. I still feel a slight tinge of embarrassment recalling the time when he asked me where I'd picked up the word "cool" from. Until he asked, I'd never considered that I'd picked the word up from anyone. I was thirteen and was quickly attempting to form my own identity and represent a particular style—something that said "grown up" and, well, "cool." But when I looked back at the conversation we'd just had, I'd used "cool" in just about every sentence. I was using the word more like a comma than a descriptor. This conversation had me begin considering how each word we say is an act of creation in and of itself, which I got to think a lot more about once I went to university as an English major. But that was years to come.

If I describe a meal that's been cooked for me, for example, as "OK" but what I mean is it's "delicious" or that I loved the bright lemony notes of the dish, then I am creating an impression with the person that I'm talking to, possibly the person who actually cooked the meal, that is not accurate. This could affect us both in any number of ways: the next time they cook for me they may feel less enthusiastic about it, they may think I didn't enjoy their cooking, or they may think the dish itself was bad. But, if I had been specific from the beginning, the results would have been entirely different.

The reason I have focused on language is because being deliberate with your communications is an important part of sensuality. In the next section, I'll define sensuality and how this term fits into the larger idea of how sensuality and sexuality are different.

What is sensuality?

First, let me start by saying that sensuality has kind of a bad rap in our culture. The *Oxford English Dictionary* defines "sensual" much in the way that you'd guess: pertaining to the senses. But, as the *OED* tends to do, there is a fuller definition that I don't think we always consider when using this word:

> Involving gratification of the senses; of, relating to, or arising from physical (esp. sexual) urges or desires and not the intellect or spirit; carnal, fleshly, base. In more neutral sense: relating to, characterized by, or involving enjoyment derived from the senses; physically enjoyable or pleasurable.[1]

In the first sentence, that oddly negative connotation is evident from the words "base" and "carnal" and also in the way that sensuality is put in opposition to intellect. Who is to say our use of the senses are not having to do with the intellect, for surely, we could not enjoy our senses without use of our brains, the source of intellect?

In addition, the *OED* mentions the association with sexuality. For many, the two words are used nearly interchangeably. Often sensuality is used merely as a softer, mood-lit version of sexuality. There's a silk-sheets and red-roses mystique attached to the word that has more to do with advertising, as far as I can tell. Through the *Huffington Post*, you can decide if you're "Sexy, Sensual or Intimate—What Is Your Sexual Style?"[2] and through *Cosmopolitan*, you can "Uncover Your Sensual Side: Enhance Your Own Pleasure and Have Him Groveling for More!"[3] Both subjects associate the word sensual with sexuality or with sex itself, which is quite commonplace. The word is frequently used as an outright marketing gimmick. I found from a quick Google search that the word "sensual" is used to sell everything from lip gloss[4] to wigs[5] to massage oil.[6]

But I was raised understanding this word in a different way. It's a word that was defined for me in the way we prepared food, cleaned the house, and got dressed for dinner. I saw it in the way my mom and dad kissed goodnight and in the way we resolved arguments in our regular house meetings. It was evident in most aspects of our decision making, planning, and in our individual communications to one another.

Sensuality is about paying attention to your senses. We have five senses through which to experience the universe: taste, touch, sight, sound, and smell, and we also have "conceptual thought," our mind or what we think about. A sixth sense, not just an M. Night Shyamalan movie from the nineties. We are sensing beings.

For me, sensuality is more of a mindset than it is a "Sexual Style," in the words of *Huffington Post*. Paying attention to your senses requires being in the present moment. Often, we can get caught up thinking about what is to come, the future, or what has already happened, the past. But I've found that when I'm living my life in present time, I'm taking in what's around me in that very moment. I don't think about how the place I'm in reminds me of when I was a kid, or how I wished it looked different. I see that place as it is and without value. It's the most effective way to enjoy your life on a daily basis.

Here's a practical way of thinking about this: ever since I was in college, I have loved a good cup of tea. It started as a way to warm up during long hours of sitting and reading and also as a minor procrastination while getting work done. If I was stuck midway through getting a thought out, I could always spring up mid-sentence and make a cup of tea and stretch my legs for a moment. It certainly looked (and felt) a lot better than checking Facebook for the hundredth time. This tea habit eventually grew into a practice and I found that I enjoyed the entire ritual of making tea, from boiling the water to swirling the final dregs in the bottom of my cup. It's a pause, a moment in my day that results in something so simple yet infinitely pleasurable.

My sister makes ceramics and our cupboard is filled to the brim with an assortment of hand-thrown mugs of porcelain and Black Mountain and red clay with varying glazes ranging from pure creamy-white to a soft gray-blue. I don't have a particular favorite as I have many favorites instead. I relish the ones with a soft rim from the thick pour of the glaze. I savor the rough sides that remain unglazed and rub against my fingertips like a large-grain emery board. Each cup has a quirk, a bald spot where it was burned clean in the kiln firing, or a misshaping to the circular barrel of the vessel. That's why we have them in our cupboards, because of their little eccentricities. Each morning, I get to choose the one that feels the best to me: I can pick a quirk that matches me.

Heating up the cup with quick swirls of boiling water results in a cup of tea at the temperature that I prefer, so I take that extra step first thing. Our tea shelf is bursting with a variety of tea from savory herbal all the way to a peculiar "extra-caffeinated" caramel black tea, which everyone in the house seems to avoid. Loose-leaf Earl Grey is my preference and I have sought out the perfect blend that provides the right balance of bitter tea and perfumey-bergamot. Not too floral, not too bubble-gum, but bold enough to announce "Earl Grey" with confidence. Covering the tea cup, I leave it to steep for about four minutes. Any longer and the black tea takes over and makes the whole thing become too bold, which is a bit heavy for first thing in the morning. But if I rush it and take the tea out too soon, the tea is lackluster and when I add the milk—it looks too milky and unappealing. If I steep it just right, the milk looks like a rich caramel in my cup.

Standing at the kitchen sink, I take in the orchids that crowd our window box. Each bloom reaching out and declaring "hello" with it's bright, round face. Their long stems wind through the various pots and containers and filter the morning sunlight. The cup is hot in my hands and the steam warms my chest. That first sip says so much—the right amount of tea, the right amount of milk, and that bitter kick that makes my lips purse just the slightest.

This is a form of sensuality; it's taking in all that is around you. I'm going to make tea first thing in the morning because I like the caffeine boost but, with each cup I make each morning, I have the choice every step of the way to make it a sensual experience. Alternatively, I could rush into the kitchen, grab the first cup that I saw, give it a quick rinse to slough out any leftover debris from the previous use, fill it with hot water, and drop a Lipton tea bag in there and be on my way. Plenty of mornings look like that and I still leave the kitchen having produced the necessary cup of tea. But when I do take those steps with the kind of attention that I described, I feel different; it makes a difference in my body. There is often a solidity and a calm that comes with being deliberate and creating pleasure in any given moment.

Before we go further, I want to bring particular attention to an aspect of that tea time I described, which is being deliberate. This is a way of being that will crop up frequently in this book in ways that are both direct (by using the actual word) and indirect (describing a moment in which this concept is occurring). For me, it's a central aspect of sensuality. To be deliberate means to fully consider and have intention with what you are doing, a key part of being deliberate is having attention on what is happening.[7] This concept is often associated with going slowly, which is part of being deliberate but is not necessarily intrinsic to the way I understand it. Having attention and using your intention are the two main components of being deliberate.

What is sexuality?

Sexuality is all about reproduction, or activities relating to reproducing the species. In this context, I use the word "sexual" to *only* describe activities or experiences that are about reproduction. This way of understanding the word "sexuality" underlines a larger concept about goals. Reproduction is a goal-oriented idea: the goal is to reproduce the species.

There is nothing wrong with sexuality, we are all here as the result of a successful sexual act. However, when it comes to human reproduction there is no female orgasm required in sexual acts. Instead, the focus is all about male orgasm because that's the only orgasm during intercourse that is required to make the babies. Hence, sexuality is a goal-oriented word.

There's nothing wrong with being goal-oriented. Goals are good, it's how we get things done. I set goals for myself every day, each year, and throughout my conversations; I am constantly picking up other goals that I want to have from relating to my friends. The reason I am making the distinction about "goal-orientation" is that it can limit the experiences we have because we get so focused on the end result. Instead of the experience I described before that involved all of my senses in making a hot beverage for myself, it's more like just pouring some hot water and plopping a tea bag in. It'll be hot, it'll be brewed, and it'll be in a cup—that's all you know for sure. With the previous example, I took pleasure from each aspect of the experience leading up to making the cup, consuming it, and enjoying how I felt afterwards. Since the process in and of itself was pleasurable, the tea itself is more of an addition—it's not the only important component. With a goal-oriented mindset, the tea (or the end result) is the most important part. If the tea is no good, or whatever result you were expecting doesn't happen, then the whole experience is bad.

What I'm describing here is actually two different ways of looking at life: a pleasure-oriented perspective or a goal-oriented perspective, also referred to as production-oriented. Most people go through life looking at the production aspects: getting a good job, getting a house, finding a partner, etcetera. That's a good way of doing things because all of those aspects of life are excellent: I want people to live in homes, have jobs, and live happily ever after with someone that they love. But what I'm pointing out here, and what I'll be exploring in this book, is how to incorporate a pleasure-oriented perspective into our lives. It's an addition, not a total change of course.

Connected to this distinction between pleasure-orientation and production-orientation, as demonstrated in the difference between sensuality and sexuality, is a concept that I learned about once I was an adult doing my own research about human sexuality. The concept is called "two levels of awareness," which is the idea that two views or ideas about one thing can both be true at the same time. This is perhaps best illustrated by a table. If you touch your desk or whatever flat surface you happen to be near, it'll be solid against your fingertips. But at the same time, it's comprised of a whirling mass of atoms on a microscopic level. Even though this is true, the table will still hold up whatever you set upon it, like your water glass or cup of tea. Both of these views about a table are correct, even if they seem to contradict one another.

It's a different way of looking at the views we have about the people and ideas in our lives. We're typically taught that there is one *right* way of thinking about a thing, but in reality, there are hundreds if not thousands of perspectives on any given issue or experience. Being able to hold more than one viewpoint at a time is not only possible, but it's imperative if you want to have a broader perspective, especially when it comes to sensuality.

Why? Because I'm not asking you to change anything that you're already doing, I'm only asking for you to consider another viewpoint. What I said earlier about a production-oriented viewpoint and a pleasure-oriented viewpoint is not my attempt to demolish the way you and everyone else lives. What I'm actually seeking is balance, a bit more pleasure with the production. A little more sensuality with the sexuality.

Why? Because it's integral to having comprehensive, sex-positive conversations about our personal choices, our bodies, and how we relate to our partners. So often conversations around sexuality stop at the mechanics instead of talking about the foundation, about what comes first. And this idea of two levels of awareness is one of the fundamental viewpoints I use when it comes to expanding my own life. It's a viewpoint, a tool even, that will come in handy throughout this book and the ideas explored within it.

Throughout this book I'll be returning to these fundamental concepts: sensuality, pleasure-orientation, and using specific language. My goal is to provide another way of looking at aspects of life that we're all going to experience at some point: growing up, growing bodies, engaging in sexual activity, and communicating, to name a few. In the next chapter we'll look at how a pleasure-oriented view changes the way a person views his or her own body.

Part 1

Exploring the Body

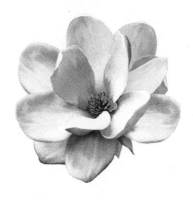

Chapter 2

ANATOMY WITH
AN EMPHASIS ON PLEASURE

Like a lot of kids, while growing up I liked learning how to dance. I took all kinds of dance classes; from hip-hop classes in the Mission District of San Francisco to an occasional ballet class in the then-small town of Redding, to a year or so of jazz classes. Through that training, I began to learn how people memorize different kinds of movement and learn from one another. My first public performance was a wreck in the way that little kids' performances often are: on stage, I confronted the fact that even though I'd been to all the practices and done all the rehearsals, I hadn't actually learned the steps. My trick of watching the other girls and copying what they did didn't work anymore because now they were dancing all over the place and I couldn't keep up. My experience of that "performance" was mainly me floundering around from side to side on a brightly lit stage in front of an auditorium of strangers while dressed in my adorable black jumpsuit with rainbow-stripe side-detailing. It was a disorienting and strange experience; I don't think I was even old enough to be embarrassed. It didn't matter, anyways, as my entire family greeted me after the performance with huge, welcoming smiles and hugs.

I learned the most about dancing in our living room. While my sister and I were growing up, dance parties and performances were a big part of how we'd celebrate. Every New Year's Eve most of my community would pull together to create a group skit that Sophia and I would write and organize, and people would pick songs to sing or dance to or prepare a performance of whatever talent they wanted to show off. I knew that these parties were a lot of fun and I would frequently put one on myself, regardless of whether or not it was a holiday. Usually I'd spend a few days practicing a dance (I'd mainly practice to get familiar with the music) and then would choose an evening to perform, sometime after dinner but before all of us dispersed to do dishes and head to bed.

Without much preamble, I'd put the song on and then just start dancing. I'd feel the attention of my audience, my family and best friends, and then would move however it suited me. I had a small repertoire of dance moves from my jazz or hip-hop classes, or movements I'd seen the grown-ups use at our dance parties that I'd like but would mainly just do what I felt. I'd hear the music and shift and bounce and undulate to the beats and just do what I wanted. Whenever I looked at my dad or mom, I would feel their approval and their enjoyment.

There was one particularly fun night that stands out when I was nine years old. I'd picked a song that I really liked, Whitney Houston's "My Love Is Your Love" from the album of the same name. The song had come out recently and, as a second-generation Whitney Houston fan, I was into it. I felt it in that particular way you sometimes do, where the song somehow rests in your body when you hear it: it clicks, it's right. I knew this was a song worth performing to and I had choreographed a set of steps to begin the dance that involved several long, slow steps out into the middle of the room along with the steady, sultry beat of the beginning of the song. It was big for me to memorize steps, since as I mentioned earlier it wasn't really intuitive for me. But I'd done it: I had a plan and an outfit (which was a pair of stretchy navy-blue jazz pants and a red halter that coordinated in that special way that clothes only do on a nine year old).

That night was a hit: after those four minutes and twenty-one seconds had elapsed everyone stood up and clapped and a huge surge of energy washed over me. Their approval was like a wave crashing over my tiny frame and I loved the thrill of being swept up in it. I ran over to my dad and gave him a hug and kiss and then found my mom and snuggled up to her, infinitely pleased with myself and what I'd created.

The next day, I decided I wanted to do it again. This time, we were going to record it on our handheld VHS camcorder. After dinner once more, I put on the song and I did my steps, this time in a different outfit (a white-crocheted halter with bright purple daisies appliquéd to the front). I tried to recreate what I'd done last night: I began with the same slow, lengthy steps diagonally across the room, stopping in the center just as Whitney's voice changed the direction of the song, but this time it was different. I couldn't wait for the song to be over because I just didn't feel right. Afterward when I looked up, there was my loving audience, just as before, but I could tell they knew. Of course, they still hugged me and loved me just like last time, but I felt slightly put off.

Later on, my dad asked me if the two performances had been the same and I told him, no, they were not. I acknowledged that I'd felt different this time and realized that it was just that, the feeling. I hadn't let myself get swept up in the music as I had the first time. That song is emotional and rich and when I danced the first time I felt like I got to express the intent of the message through my own movement. But the second time around I'd tried to replicate my success of the previous evening: memorization over simply doing what I felt.

As we get older, girls are taught to value looking good over feeling good. We're expected to show up at our jobs and look and act a certain way regardless of what's going on in our lives. But in order to live a pleasurable life, it's more important to value feeling good. What I learned most from the myriad of dance performances for my family is to value feeling. I felt firsthand the difference between when I was enjoying what I was doing and when I was just going through the motions. They approved of me no matter what; I got cheers and hugs regardless of what I went up there and did. But the times when I went out there and let myself out, when I felt the music and let it roll through and out of me, that's when I knew people could feel me being me.

From my view, the first step to valuing how you feel over how you look is being confident in what you've got. For the rest of this chapter, we will explore different aspects of the human body from a pleasurable perspective. Often when we are taught about human sexuality we mainly learn about the reproductive aspects of our bodies. But reproduction is a small part of who we are and what we're capable of. The ability to reproduce is quite limited for women (or those with uteri and the accompanying reproductive parts) as women have a finite period of time during their lives in which they can have babies, should they even decide to do so at all. Many people choose not to reproduce or are physically unable to do so. But meanwhile, what everyone *does* have are sensational areas of their body which can bring them pleasure. These parts may be different for different people, but in this chapter we'll explore some of the main areas just to get you started. This chapter concludes with two different exercises you can do yourself to get you going in your own full-body pleasure-seeking explorations.

Before I go any further, it's important to acknowledge that not everyone experiences their genitalia the way that is depicted in the drawings which follow or in the words I've used so far or will use. Gender is a fluid concept, more like a spectrum than the binary that we are usually taught. The descriptions of genitalia may or may not correspond to your own or your specific gender identity, which I respect. I have done my best to use language which is inclusive as my aim is to further our education of one another's bodies so that we can all be happier and experience more pleasure in our lives.

The Brain

How we experience pleasure actually has very little do with our genitalia. All pleasure begins conceptually, which is good news because while our bodies vary greatly in terms of size, shape, ability, and form, a commonality is our minds. Heather Corinna, sex educator and author, describes the brain and its structures as the "the largest, most important and most active sexual organ of the body."[1] Our brain is responsible for the running of our various systems (like the cardiovascular system, for example) and our hormones. Our minds are also where we create emotions and is the harbor of our personal preferences. It's the place where we process the input from our senses, including touch, taste, sight, and all the rest. Without our brains there would be no pain or pleasure, just as there would be no orgasm, since the brain is the head of our nervous system.

Learning what you enjoy is a distinct pleasure of its own, because your preferences and pleasure are unique from anyone else's. We all experience our senses differently and, based on our own life experiences and values, have different likes and dislikes. Time and experience can affect our preferences, so just because you liked one thing yesterday doesn't mean you'll like the same thing today. Just as the brain is the place where we process the input from our senses, it's also the place where we store all of our back story: the past experiences we've had, the ways other people have interacted with us or taught us, and the choices and decisions we've made for ourselves. All of this can affect the way we view our own bodies and experience pleasure, for better or for worse.

Skin and Hair

Pleasure can be experienced in any number of ways through any number of body parts: our whole bodies are available. Our skin is our largest organ and weighs from six to ten pounds on average. Rich with nerve endings and receptors, almost every part of the skin is covered with fine sensory nerves.[2] How sensational each part of our skin is ranges from area to area (and person to person!) but, generally speaking, areas with hair are more sensitive to pressure and our skin is thinner in areas were hair does not grow. Take a look for yourself: the skin on the backs of your knees or hands may feel like a different texture or thickness than that of your scalp or armpits. Areas that grow hair tend to be more sensitive due to the increase in sense receptors at the base of each hair.[3] Diane Ackerman, in her marvelous book on our capacity to sense, *A Natural History of the Senses*, points out the complexity of the hairs we grow and how they affect our ability to sense:

> One hair can easily be triggered: If something presses or tugs at it, if its tip is touched [. . .] Still, it can't be firing all the time, or the body would go into sensory overload. There is an infinitesimally small realm is which nothing at all seems to be happening, a desert of sensation. Then the merest breeze starts to blow, nothing like a real disturbance. When it grows just strong enough to reach an electrical threshold, it fires an impulse to the nervous system. Hairs make wonderful organs of touch.[4]

Not just our skin, but the very hairs we are covered with, from the finest to the thickest or curliest, are filled with potential for sensation.

There are parts of our bodies that are particularly sensitive and sometimes referred to as *erogenous zones* or areas with erectile tissue (tissue where blood flow increases the available sensation). Examples of this are lips, nipples, and genitals. Our sensitive lips, tongues, and genitals all have neural receptors called Krause end bulbs and thus "similarity of response" of all of these areas.[5] Other sensitive areas are necks, breasts, inner thighs, or any area which *you* find sensational. Some people take enjoyment from the inside of their elbows, which is to say that you have free rein over your own body to find the areas that are sensitive and sensational for you.[6]

Hands

For the most part, our hands are our most dexterous, agile body parts. And although they are not usually thought of as part of our pleasurable toolbox, I would certainly say they belong there. Our hands are dense with nerve endings, which contributes to our ability for fine motor control (most easily seen with the use of tools). Our hands are a dexterous wonderment of receptors and nerve endings which allow for this body part to communicate with our brains incredibly well. Our fingertips are particularly sensitive: through them we can detect changes in temperature, texture, and shape without the use of sight. Try running your fingertips across this page or on any surface near you without looking and see what information you can gather in such a simple motion. Our hands are a form of "antennae" for our bodies: the palms alone are home to seventeen thousand touch receptors and nerve endings which are capable of perceiving pressure, movement, and vibration.[7] This ability is a great contributor to our ability to seek and experience pleasurable aspects of our lives.[8]

Breasts and Nipples

Breasts and nipples can be highly sensational areas of our bodies, whether or not we develop full-on breasts (typically, those with testes develop very little breast matter). One of the earliest forms of development in puberty, breast changes are often referred to as "budding" because it can feel like a small bud, akin to a flower bud, developing under the nipple. This doesn't necessarily mean it will happen at the same time, development is sometimes asymmetric, which is just fine and nothing to worry about. Changes will steadily occur to the nipple area

(called the "areola") and surrounding breast tissue. And, breasts continue changing throughout people's lifetimes. Weight fluctuation, menstruation, pregnancy,
and sexual activity are just a few factors that can affect the size or sensation of
your breasts. There is a lot of variation in breasts: size, shape, location, and nipple
size/color/shape/location. Just about every aspect of a breast can vary from person to person and breast to breast. No two breasts are perfectly alike, even on the
same person! Which, in my opinion, is a big part of what makes breasts so fun.[9]

If you have a uterus, your breasts contain mammary glands (called "lobules")
and milk-carrying ducts. Breasts contain no muscle; they're comprised of fat
and glands. There is muscle beneath the breast itself, which can affect the shape
of the breast. The darker, more textured skin closer to the center of the breast is
called the areola, which then leads to the nipple. Hormone levels can alter breast
size and shape within any given month, but the main determining factor is
genetics.[10]

For those without a uterus, your breasts and nipples will change during
puberty as well, although not as dramatically. Usually a nipple "bud" develops,
which can feels like a hardening under the nipple itself.[11] Regardless of your
breast situation, you'll have nipples.

Nipples can be highly sensitive areas for all kinds of bodies. Occasionally
nipples appear more as an "inny" than an "outy," which is not usually a cause
for concern: 10–20 percent of people have inverted nipples.[12]

Breasts and nipples can also be hairy. Hair isn't necessarily determined by the
sex of the person, either. It has more to do with genetics, just as everything else
having to do with breasts does. People don't talk a lot about nipple hair, but it's
certainly a real thing and nothing to be troubled by. In fact, hair around the
nipples could be an added sensory delight since hairs are an indicator of sensory
receptors, as was discussed in the section on skin and hair.

Vulva

The "vulva" describes all of the external parts of female genitalia and includes
the *mons* (the upper area of soft, padded tissue resting on top of the pubic bone
where the majority of pubic hair is located), *labia majora* (the thicker, outer lips,

which are often covered in part by pubic hair), *labia minora* (the second set of lips that are within, which may be larger or smaller than the outer labia majora), *clitoris* (often covered by a *clitoral hood* which can vary in size), *urethral opening* (located below the clitoris but above the opening to the vagina, this is the hole where urine exits the body), and the entrance to the vagina, or *introitus*. Please refer to the accompanying drawing for an introduction to where these parts are located.[13]

There are many sensational parts to a vulva. The mons itself is rich with

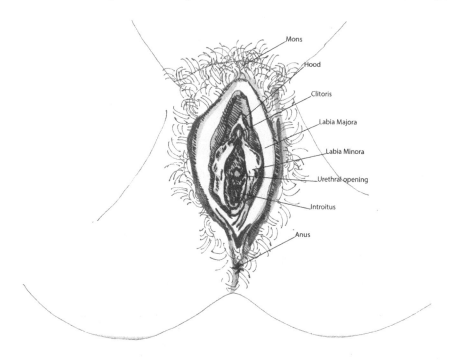

nerve endings and the presence of pubic hair can add to our capacity for experiencing sensation. Located further down, just under a peak of skin called the hood, is the clitoris which is chock-full of nerve endings and has enormous potential for sensation. So much so that the clitoris gets its own section in this chapter. The labia themselves are also sensational.[14]

While much emphasis is put on vaginas as being key to vulvar pleasure, that's mainly a myth. Most of what is sensational inside the vagina is due to the clitoris being fully engorged (conversely, if not engorged, those sensational parts won't be available). Most of the nerve endings in the vagina are located around the opening, also called the introitus. In fact, the back two-thirds of the vagina (the part closest to the cervix, the entrance to the uterus) has almost no nerve endings at all and is not sensitive to fine touch. Fine touch is the detail-rich touch that we can feel on our hands, thighs, and other nerve-ending rich parts of our bodies (like our clitorises!). The majority of nerve endings exist in the remaining third of the vagina closest to the entrance, and in this area the internal part of the clitoris, perineum (the sensation-dense area between the introitus and the anus), and urethral sponge (an area located toward the entrance of the vagina, which some people find sensational) are all located, which have great potential for pleasurable sensation.[15]

The size, amount of sensation, and location will vary from vulva to vulva. As with all parts of our bodies, there is enormous variety in not only how we look, but how we feel. There is no need to compare your genitals with another person's, because each is unique. I highly recommend checking out Heather Corinna's online work (scarletteen.org) as she has an excellent article on variations in vulvas[16] and I also recommend looking up the famed sex researcher Betty Dodson's book *Sex for One** as she has done much to illuminate the range of lovely vulvas in the world.[17]

Clitoris

I have a lot to say about the clitoris, so please take a seat. First of all, we're not the only animals who have them. All female mammals have a clitoris which means that your neighbor's pet puppy, the monkeys at the zoo, and most farm animals all have something in common. Whether or not all animals experience pleasure is the subject of debate, but several primates, including our close cousins the bonobo, have been observed experiencing female orgasm.[18]

Depending on the animal, the clitoris comes in many shapes and sizes, but a commonality is that the sole purpose of the clitoris is for pleasure. One interesting exception to this is the spotted hyena, which urinates and gives birth

---

* The resources of this text contain the URL of an article version of *Sex for One* which contains reproductions of the illuminating images I refer to as well as a link to Corinna's article on vulva variation.

through her clitoris.[19] I think it's good to keep in mind that we're all part of the animal kingdom: our bodily functions, including our pleasure, are not anything particularly special to humans. So, since we happen to be one of the many animals with a clit, why not celebrate it?

The word "clitoris" stems from the Greek "*kleitoris*," meaning "little hill."[20] And for centuries, people have thought of the clitoris that way and consequently have grown to believe that the female glans for pleasure is hidden, small, or difficult to access. But we now know, publicly, that it's much more than that (although, between you and me, many people have known for a long time that there is a lot more going on with the clitoris than just a "little hill"). In 2005, Dr. Helen O'Connell published the first-ever comprehensive research on the internal aspects of the clitoris,[21] which completely changed the conversation we are able to have about women's ability to feel pleasure.

O'Connell's MRI scans demonstrated that the clitoris is not just the glans we can see externally, but is actually made up of several different parts, all of which are comprised of erectile tissue. Erectile tissue means that these areas engorge with blood during arousal.

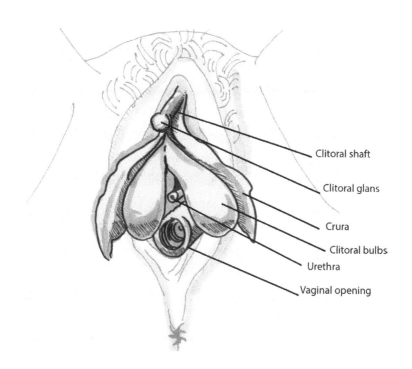

Clitoral shaft

Clitoral glans

Crura

Clitoral bulbs

Urethra

Vaginal opening

In this illustration, we can see the entire structure of the clitoris including the glans (the external portion), crura (the longer "legs" of the clitoris), and the clitoral bulbs. All of these parts make up the structure of the clitoris and expands earlier notions of the clitoris which considered the clitoris to only be the external portion.[22]

• • • • • •

The clitoris is the only organ of the body (either female or male) that is solely dedicated to pleasure. The only function of the clitoris is to feel: we do not urinate, have babies, or defecate from our clitoris. Many other parts of our bodies have nerve endings which can be taken advantage of for our pleasure, but the clitoris is the only one that's just there for our own enjoyment. The clitoris can be very sensitive: there are over eight-thousand pressure sensitive nerve endings in the glans, which is a relatively small surface area in the external portion of the vulva. The penis has just as many nerve endings, but they're spread out over the glans and shaft of the penis. To that point, the glans of the clitoris has a concentration of nerve endings fifty times that of the penis.[23]

Sexologist Mal Harrison created her own sonogram images of the structure of the clitoris and has worked to expand our collective education about the full extent of the clitoris, not just the part visible from the outside of the body.[24]

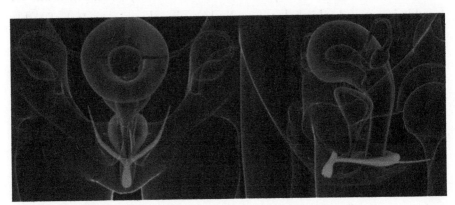

Images courtesy of Mal Harrison, Center for Erotic Intelligence

In this graphic, we can see the internal structure of the clitoris in relation to the pubic bone and vaginal opening. This internal portion is shaped much like that of a wishbone. Learning the full extent of this organ is important for our own understanding of what our bodies are capable of so that we are fully able to seek and experience our capacity for pleasure. These images and vocabulary are meant to serve as a starting guide for your own discovery and exploration, whether you have a clitoris yourself or care for people who do. Knowing our own bodies and that of the people we function with, whether or not it's in a sensual capacity, is key to living a fulfilled life. I am a firm believer that pleasure is our birthright.

Penis

We can divide the anatomy of the penis and testes into three main parts: the testicles, penile shaft, and head of the penis. At the head of the penis is the urethral opening: the urethra runs the length of the penis inside of the shaft and is where fluids exit the body (namely: pre-ejaculate, semen, and urine). The head of the penis, often referred to as the glans, is where the highest concentration of nerve endings in the penis reside.[25] This area may or may not be covered by a foreskin. The foreskin is a nerve-rich area of skin that, when the penis is flaccid, partly or fully covers the head of the penis. The foreskin is a self-lubricating area, which means it should slide back easily by itself or by hand. Sometimes the foreskin is removed at birth due to medical or cultural reasoning. If the foreskin has been removed, there will most likely be a small V-shaped scar or banded scar. The testes (testicles) are covered by a scrotum (an exterior covering of the testes which is comprised of skin and muscle and is usually covered with hair) and usually contain two testes.[26] The testes are where testosterone and sperm are produced.[27]

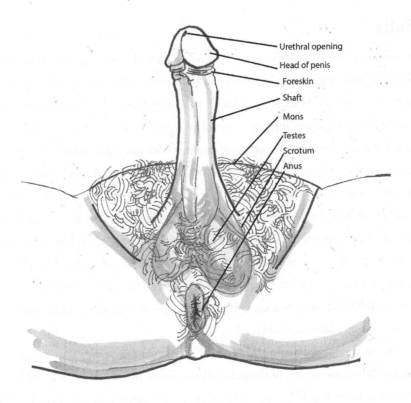

Urethral opening
Head of penis
Foreskin
Shaft
Mons
Testes
Scrotum
Anus

The penis is made up of three main cylinders of tissue which run its length. These cylinders are the *corpora cavernosa* (of which there are two) and the *corpus spongiosum*. These cylinders are what fill with blood when a penis gets erect (so, no, in case you were wondering there is no actual bone in a penis).[28] Erections can (and do) occur from infancy throughout the rest of life, although the ability to ejaculate arrives during puberty.[29] Interestingly, the clitoris is comprised of similar cylinders which get erect in much the same way as a penis, but instead of happening outside of the body, the engorgement mainly happens internally.[30]

Of course, as with the rest of the topics covered in this chapter, there is a lot more to say about the penis and the testes. The purpose of this section is to lay out the basics and get the ball rolling with your own research. For more information, please refer to chapter 4 on menustration where I cover more about our reproductive aspects. For further information, check out Heather Corinna's excellent sex ed book, *S.E.X.* Your health provider will also be able to provide more information about the anatomy of the penis and surrounding genital area.

Butts

And last but not least, we've got our butts! Which, despite all the cultural stigma that you may or may not be aware of about butts, they can be quite the sensational areas of our bodies. As with all our body parts, there's nothing gross or wrong about experiencing any kind of pleasure from a particular area, and in fact, the anus contains a lot of nerve endings with great potential for pleasurable sensation,[31] so why not take advantage of that? There are all sorts of ways to take pleasure from this area of our bodies, not just through penetration. Strokes, touches, or just checking it out visually to see what it looks like can all be pleasurable. Enjoying your butt says nothing about your sexual preferences, orientation, or identity. The only thing that kind of experience indicates is that you are taking advantage of what your body has to offer. Please note that the anus does not self-lubricate, so if you are going to experiment with touch make sure to use some kind of additional lubrication.

Due to the musculature and how the assortment of nerves that encircles the anus connects to the rest of the pelvic floor, this is an area that can be felt during sensual activity regardless of whether or not it's being touched directly. When experiencing contractions due to arousal or during climax, many of the nerves and muscles that are located in this area are stimulated. Located near the anus is the perineum. For those with vulvas, it's the strip in between the opening to the vagina and the anus, sometimes referred to as the perineal sponge. This area is part of the clitoral network of nerves and is comprised of erectile tissue. For those with penises, this area is also referred to as the perineum and is also an area associated with a network of nerves.[32]

In regard to those with penises, in this area is also the prostate. The prostate is a walnut-sized gland that is located in between the base of the penis and the rectum (for a visual aid please refer to the previous drawing of the anatomy of the penis, and also the drawing on page 52 which illustrates the internal anatomy of those with a penis). Although this area cannot be seen from outside the body, it can be felt by pressing either the perineal area or by penetrating the anus. Although the prostate contributes to the production of semen, I mention it here because it's a sensation-rich area that is largely what makes anal sex enjoyable. Whether or not this area is stimulated directly, the prostate contributes to sexual response.[33]

Homologous Anatomy

Now that we've delved into some of the more sensational areas of our bodies, I'd like to tell you about the ways in which genitalia are actually quite similar, despite how different they appear at first glance. In her compelling TEDx Talk, "Cliteracy" artist and educator Sophia Wallace describes the complete anatomy of the clitoris and goes on to illuminate the similarities between the penis and the clitoris in terms of shape, anatomy, and structure. She states, "our differences are not a sign of opposition, in fact, we're related to each other, we're connected, and that's an exciting fact."[34] I appreciate her point that instead of focusing on our differences, there is much to be learned from the ways we are similar.

For the first ten weeks of development, all human embryos are undifferentiated in terms of sex or gender.[35] Once certain hormones kick in, the genitalia of the embryo begin to transition into either a penis or a clitoris, but until that development we're all essentially the same.[36] This accounts for the similarity in our genitalia as adults. While from the outset the penis may look entirely different than the vulva, there are more similarities than you might imagine. In utero, the genitals form either a penis or a clitoris, genital tissues usually form scrotum (the skin surrounding the testes) or outer labia (the lips framing the outer part of the vulva), and the gonads usually either shift to become testes or ovaries.[37] This is simply an overview of the homologous nature of human genitalia and is a subject which certainly deserves more consideration. But for the purposes of this book, know that I have found that a similarity of tissue connotes a similarity in the way it may be touched and pleasurably enjoyed.

Exercises for Anatomy with an Emphasis on Pleasure

Now that we've taken time to learn about our bodies and our own capacity for pleasurable sensation, it's time to delve a bit further. Self-exploration is the best way to acquire knowledge about your body. You can figuratively build a library of yourself; each book a sensation or stroke you enjoy. There are two exercises that I highly recommend for gaining this particular kind of self-knowledge. But first, you should know about the "researcher's cap."

Before you begin these exercises, put on your researcher's cap. This means deliberately deciding to operate from the viewpoint of research. *Merriam-Webster* has defined research as: "a careful or diligent search, a studious inquiry or examination, and the collecting of information about a particular subject." We can approach our bodies in the same way: collecting information, examining, and searching. Researching means to look and simply see what you see; without attaching negative or positive judgment to your observations. It may be difficult at the beginning to look at your body without any internal critiques running through your mind, but it is possible to do so, and, with practice, it gets easier.

These exercises are an opportunity to both look at and touch your body in a deliberate way. Prior to starting, take a moment to set up your space. Ensure that you have privacy and that you won't be interrupted. You can put a note on your door if you live in a shared space, or simply lock your door. Turn your cell phone off as well as any other devices that may call out for your attention. This is a deliberate time just for you, so take a moment to ensure your peace and safety. You can also take a few moments to put on some of your favorite music and add anything else to the space that will add to your enjoyment. If you like candles, light some. If you have a beverage you enjoy, take a moment to prepare it for yourself just the way you like it. Then you will be ready to begin.

Part One

First, start with a visual inventory. If you have a small hand-mirror and a full-length mirror available, that is ideal. Using both will allow you to look at places you may have never seen before. Have you ever looked at the top of your own head, for example?

When you begin your visual inventory, do so with a non-judgmental eye. Remember, this is research and since it's research, you're looking and you're not placing value. If you find that you start criticizing, just decide to stop. You can cut off that train of thought as soon as it begins and instead choose your "researcher's cap." Placing value doesn't add to this exercise and it will only limit your experience of your body.

I recommend doing this exercise naked. Think of this as a great opportunity to see what you're working with as this is designated time to do nothing except check yourself out. Use your hand-mirror to look at your back, the backs of your knees, the bottoms of your feet. Explore your body as you see fit. It can be fun to look at different body parts up close. This is also an excellent opportunity to look at your genitals. Try bending over in front of the mirror, for example. I remember the first time I did this as an adult, I was really fascinated and surprised by what I saw. It's strange to think that while your body is something that you use every day, you may not know exactly what it looks like. Try laying back on your bed or couch and opening your legs. Use your hand mirror to see what's there. Everyone's genitals are unique and there is no "right" or "wrong" way to look. Vulvas and penises come in all shapes, sizes, and colors. It's worth finding out what yours looks like since it's totally unique.

Part Two

The next exercise is an opportunity to touch your body deliberately. This is a time to touch your body and find out what you like. You can do this while you're still lying down, seated, or in whatever comfortable position works for you. Touch your body using a "taking touch," that is, do what feels good to your hand. If you were to touch velvet, you wouldn't do it in a way to try to affect a response from the velvet. You touch it in a way that feels best to your hand. You can touch yourself and others in the same way.

Take this time to stroke your whole body: from your head to your toes. Vary the pressure and speed as you touch. Pick an area to experiment with different pressures, like your abdomen for example. Figure out what pressure or stroke you like best in that moment. What you like may change and vary day by day, so this is an excellent way to find out where you're at in the moment. Knowing what you like is an important part of being a sensual person.

Through these exercises you can train yourself to value feeling good over looking good. I first learned about these methods of exploring my body when I was just entering puberty and I used them as a way to build my own enjoyment of myself. They were a way for me to notice different changes, whether that was more body hair in different places, variations in skin tone throughout the change in seasons, or different muscle groups that became more prominent as I exercised more during soccer and boxing practices. One time I bent over, with my back facing the mirror and was surprised to see the musculature in my butt. Before that discovery, I thought butts were mostly just blobs of skin and fat, but there were these long striations of muscles running down my back and connecting to the backs of my legs and thighs that I'd never seen before. While I'm a bit more familiar with my own anatomy now, I still use these exercises regularly to notice the changes that are still occurring as I age, take on new sports and interests, and create different experiences for myself.

We'll be discussing more about body changes throughout our lives in the following chapter. The exercises that I've just described are a key part of knowing your own body, which ties back in to my original point about our bodies: it's more important to feel good than it is to look good. Looking good is something that happens externally and is more about the show we put on for other people. Feeling good is how you feel inside, the literal feelings in your body as well as the quality of your thoughts. This will be an ongoing topic throughout this book, as feeling good is a multifaceted experience which is an integral part of leading a pleasurable life.

Chapter 3

PUBERTY, BODIES, AND, OH, THESE CHANGING TIMES

As I got out of the shower, still dripping wet and wrapped in a cloud of warm steam, I looked down and saw them. After over two years of waiting and anticipating, they had arrived. Three long, gently curled, pubic hairs. I was ecstatic and then immediately perplexed: how long had they been there, and I hadn't noticed? They seemed to have shown up overnight—where had they even come from?

I showed off this new development right away. Walking into the next room, I found my mom and whipped off my bath towel to show her. She was, of course, happy for me. I beamed in pride. But then, she took the liberty of informing Julia, who was nearly a mother to me. Word travels fast when you live in a group, you see. The next time we saw Julia, my mom asked me to show her my new development. I enthusiastically pulled down my pants to show off what I'd created, as I was still quite pleased with myself at this great accomplishment. After all, I told myself, growing body hair is an undeniable sign of womanhood, even at age eleven. But then Julia did what I'd suggest no mother-figure ever do: she called my three new pubic hairs "cute." She even called them "*so* cute" in the borderline-saccharine way that moms do when they see their offspring in princess Halloween costumes or birthday dresses. I took great offense and, naturally, stalked away, red-faced. (A word to the wise, choose your adjectives carefully when talking to any pubescent person about their body.)

Since the pubic triplets first appeared on my body, many, many more have followed. Everyone knows that adolescence brings changes, whether that's hair, breast developments, periods, or deeper voices. What no one told me was that

29

this is an experience that keeps on giving well into your twenties. For a lot of us, this is no more evident than in body hair development. Hair just keeps on growing and spreading: in my late teens I both welcomed toe hair into my life and finally acknowledged my pronounced unibrow. I realized that one stray pube had taken root on my inner thigh the other day, inches away from the rest of the flock, and causing a good deal of eye-rolling on my part.

Everyone's experience of puberty is different. Some kids, like me, are all about it. Others are much more private and keep the experience to themselves as much as possible. Some develop later than others, some earlier. One aspect of group living that I took full advantage of was asking for stories. I'd get people whom I lived with on my required daily running program (yet another perk of homeschooling!) and would query them endlessly about "firsts" of any kind. What was your first kiss like? When did you first get boobs? I wanted details. I would compare notes whenever possible (for example when my sister was willing to tell me about her personal experience) and would spy on my peers to see where they were at in their own development. I was shocked when I realized the boys on my soccer team had armpit hair because, in my mind, that meant they definitely had hair *down there,* information which I was delighted to glean.

As with most change, I've found that communication is key. Periodically, I would talk to my parents about their bodies and how they changed when entering puberty. My dad told me a story once about how when he was a kid, he poured root beer on his toes to try and get hair to grow. Not only did I find that very entertaining, but it also changed my perspective on my own toe hair. I went from feeling mild disgust to a sense of pride; it was something we both shared. Now when I see the patches of surprisingly long and wild hair gracing each of my ten toes, as well as the two extra-long hairs that randomly grow on the top of my foot, I get to think of him and smile.

But people have a range of experiences, as I said. My sister, who is one year my senior, experienced puberty quite differently. I could see her changing right before my eyes, but we rarely talked about what was going on or how either of us felt. She kept to herself as much as possible and since I had hardly any attention on her, I didn't know much of what was going on. Since we lived communally, we were always in relatively close quarters. When fifteen people share three bathrooms, you get familiar with one another quickly. We were always in rooms together, whether that was five people in a tiny kitchen prepping dinner or three people using the bathroom at once: one to pee, one to shower, and one to brush their teeth. That's the norm and it works. But somehow, Sophia made herself as invisible as humanly possible for a couple of years. I never, ever saw her completely naked. She started to dress in looser, less form-fitting clothing, and spent a lot of time in our shared bedroom by herself. Years later, I asked her about her first period and sheepishly admitted that I didn't know the story (even though I'd been right there for it). Without skipping a beat, she reminded me that I didn't know because she didn't tell me or anyone, that she hid it as well as she could.

Puberty and Body Image

Everybody experiences puberty at some point in young adulthood and it will look different for each and every one of us. Those of us with uteruses and the hormonal changes that go along with having periods experience changes that are not all that different from those with testes. Yes, on a chemical and hormonal level, the changes are quite different, but the kind of emotional growth and response to these changes (that is, how they are *experienced*) can feel quite similar. Our bodies are shifting and changing so that we are capable of reproducing and the effects of that can come out in a number of ways, including mood changes and increased sensitivity. Heather Corinna points out in her book *S.E.X.* that the hormonal changes that happen with people who have testes are cyclical in a similar way that to those that happen to people with periods. Those with testes usually experience an increase and decrease of testosterone on a twenty-four-hour cycle as well as a seventy-two-day cycle in which other hormones related to reproduction increase.[1] My point being, that despite the way our gender differences may be highlighted in popular culture, the changes we go through in development are not all that different.

Puberty is a time when we experience relatively rapid, all-over body development.[2] Our bodies continue changing throughout our lives, but the decade or so of growth that happens during puberty can be concentrated and intense.[3]

On average, puberty begins between ages eight and fourteen (although it can be later or earlier, and typically puberty begins on the earlier side for those with uteri than it does those with testes) and continues into the mid-twenties.[4] Twenty-five years old is typically the end of puberty.[5]

Generally speaking, there are a few major changes that occur during puberty. Breast development, body hair growth, all over body growth, and periods will make their appearance as well as ejaculation, skin changes, and voice changes. At the back of this book you'll find more resources for further reading about the intricacies of puberty. Some of the biggest changes are happening under our skin, however, as a myriad of hormones are at work influencing the aforementioned changes. And, at the same time, our brains are undergoing rapid development.[6] All of this change, development, and growth makes for an intense experience, which is why I believe that learning and paying attention to how our bodies *feel* as well as function are key aspects to leading more pleasurable lives. Later in this book we'll explore additional tools that speak to that point.

Body Image

Body image is "your view of your own body in function, health, experience, and appearance."[7] It includes the values you place on your appearance, your overall feelings about your entire body, from your height to your weight, and your sense of control of your body and how you feel in it.[8] Body image isn't solely about body weight and it certainly isn't just a "women's issue," as is commonly thought.[9] To put it broadly and bluntly: how you think about your body affects your experience in the world.

For further reading on the social and cultural forces that influence our perception of our body, I highly recommend the work of Sonya Renee Taylor, who founded "The Body Is Not an Apology" movement and authored a book of the same title. In her book, she explores the concept of "radical self-love," loving one's body amidst the pressures of our society. Taylor points out early on in her book that we are born enjoying our bodies exactly as they are and much of her book points to that fact. The act of enjoying ourselves for who we are begins on the inside, and the global impact that view can have, particularly spoke to me: "A radical self-love world is a world that works for every body. Creating such a world is an inside-out job. How we value and honor our bodies impacts how we value and honor bodies of others. [. . .] It is through our own transformed relationship with our bodies that we become champions for other bodies on the planet."[10]

But the truth is, I wasn't raised in a household that used the term "body image," or self-love, or radical self-love, for that matter. It's not that we avoided the topic of our bodies, or that we couldn't discuss our bodies openly. Quite the opposite; when I was a teen I frequently had conversations with my mom and friends about changes I was experiencing or how I felt about my body. It's just that we didn't use such a handy term as "body image;" instead, we were more specific, and we handled the conversation on a day-to-day basis.

. . . . . .

I stood in the mirror, glaring at my belly. Sloped, protruding, layers on layers, I wanted to glare it away. Turning to the side, I disliked the way my breasts hid behind the silhouette of my full belly. Boobs should stick out further than belly, I told myself. And look! I have pocks and lumps on my butt. As I flexed, they stood out further and I shrunk in response. The voice in my head told me all kinds of things: *I'm fourteen, this is supposed to be a time when my body looks the best it can, this is supposed to be the easiest time to be fit*, and I rattled off my laundry list of things to change. I sank myself lower and lower until I was on the verge of tears at the sight of my own body. Suddenly the door opened, and my mom entered the room. "Are you being hard on yourself?" she asked. Her presence was like a cool breeze sliding through and quieting my mind. I hadn't said a word aloud, but she felt the judgments I was having, the depths of my criticism. By asking that simple question, she gave me reality about where I was operating from. Gulping, I snapped out of it. I stopped the stream of thoughts and realized the choices that I had been making. Sure, society puts pressure on us to be thin, or muscular, or curvy or whatever, but it's my choice to listen to those voices. Looking back in the mirror, I saw my body for what it was: it's life, it's me.

Early on, I was taught the importance of approval, both of others and of myself. As humans, we place value on situations, experiences, and on each other.

It's a natural part of life and it's how we give our lives meaning. Every time, the value we place is either negative or positive (this is what I have or will refer to as a "value judgment"). Experience has no inherent value, no matter what it is. We're the ones doing the assigning and since we're going to place value anyways, it might as well be positive.

Approval of your body can be difficult when you're getting a million messages a day from the media, your peers, and possibly your parents that tell you the opposite: you're imperfect. Our culture benefits from you thinking that you're not perfect and that there is something to fix. How else would the makeup, cosmetic surgery, and weight-loss industries continue making millions?

My dad had me consider this when I was about ten years old. I had taken a shower and selected a lotion that I'd had my eye on in the cupboard for a few days. It was a small, attractive bottle of pear-scented lotion from Victoria's Secret. I'm not sure where it came from, but I distinctly remember the allure that the bottle held for me, from the light green tinge of the product, to the gold cursive that decorated the label. I rubbed it all over my body and relished the sweet, summery perfume that cloaked me.

Later that day, I saw my dad. He greeted me and rubbed my back and told me that my skin felt soft. I immediately told him all about this great lotion that I'd used, giving him an explanation for what he'd noticed. He paused and looked down at me with apparent puzzlement. He walked away, and I felt a fast sinking in my chest and wondered why he'd left. Later, I had a conversation with my mom about it and I eventually came to my conclusion: the lotion had nothing to do with it; he'd felt the softness of my skin and that was it. By adding in some kind of explanation, I had bought into the idea of this product and its ability to have an effect on me, and in turn attempted to sell it to my dad by proclaiming how well it worked.

Ultimately, it's up to you to decide how you feel about your body. There are no rules about how you should look. We're really just a bunch of meat sacks walking around on this planet, and due to genetics, it's completely arbitrary how we end up looking. Why base our happiness and self-worth on something as random as how big our noses are, or how bony our cheekbones are? It's up to you to decide how to feel about your body.

Growing up, I was never told I was pretty. It just wasn't done. Surrounded by loving adults, I was never bathed in compliments about my looks. An avid athlete, I was acknowledged for my muscular legs and my friends noticed the changes that came with long hours spent running around a soccer field. I remember my mom talking to me about how thick and at times unruly my light brown hair was. She loved to brush it, or would have if I ever let her. I was encouraged in my interests: soccer, swimming, reading, etcetera. When I felt good or happy, that's when I would get particular attention. My friends would comment on how bright my eyes were, or how fun my outfit looked. No one gushed or drew attention to my looks.

This is in sharp contrast to how we relate to most young girls. I catch myself doing this almost every time I come across a toddler. My first reaction is to tell her "how pretty" she is, or what a great dress she's wearing. I didn't even realize that this was a deliberate choice on the part of my parents until I was older when my dad told me. He mentioned, mid-conversation, that they never told us we were pretty when they were raising us. Flashing back on my life, I realized he was right. He didn't want to put that kind of pressure on us, my sister and me. And what does it matter?

That's a heavy label to throw on a woman. Prettiness has an expiration date and it comes up fast. By the time we reach mid-thirties, we're less valuable than in our teens or twenties. Prettiness is nearly as short-lived as it is narrow. While the definition is starting to expand, the standard remains: blonde, thin, blue eyes, you know the drill. And finally, your prettiness has nothing to do with you. Sure, you can color your hair and pluck your eyebrows, but it's your parents (and their parents, and the parents before them . . .) who created what you are now. If people tell me I'm pretty, I often will flicker back, mentally, to my mom and dad and silently thank *them*, because I'm a good-looking by-product of a series of their choices.

The final aspect of my training in self-confidence, my building blocks of "body image," was learning how to say, "fuck you."

We sat around our large circular dining room table and repeated those two words over and over again. My dad picked our friend Gary who sat across the table from us, and we directed the "fuck you" straight to him. It was nothing personal. I liked Gary a lot; he'd recently moved into our house and I remember that first evening we met, I ran around and under the table again and again, staring at his legs, long and bent before him, and felt completely fascinated by him as he sat at our dining room table. But this evening was different. My sister and I sat on either side of our dad and he told us to say it. If we faltered or said it too half-assed, my dad would tell us to say it again. I felt the one where I got it. There was a particular force to the words and a level of ownership that I felt in my body. Right then I learned the difference between simply saying two words and saying them with intention. I realized that I had power, that I could communicate anything I wanted, to anyone, if I decided to.

At the time I was seven and I had a buzz cut, I loved it. I'm sure I was seven because that was the year *G.I. Jane* came out and I recall touching my own buzz cut with my hand while sitting in the darkened theater watching Demi Moore shave off her hair and be a complete badass for two solid hours. Around the same time, I was having some trouble with strangers asking me "if I was a boy or a girl," as if it was any of their business. The people who asked were usually kids but very often adults would as well, with varying degrees of politeness. Once, as I was walking in the doors of our local supermarket, I let a woman pass in front of me. As she passed, she said "thank you, young man." I was dumbstruck and instantly felt hot all over my body. There she stood, nicely clad in a blue dress and wrong. So wrong. This adult who had returned my niceness with complete disregard. Later I told my Dad and he asked, "Well, did you tell her 'fuck you'?"

Rites of Passage and Growing Up

There are many rites of passage and coming of age rituals in the world and they vary by culture, geography, and the social climate itself. Examples of potential rites of passage are a quinceañera or a bar mitzvah. Some rites of passage are less structured and socially recognized: growing your first mustache as a boy might be celebrated, but ignored or covered up as a girl, for example. Generally speaking, all of our "firsts" are part of our experience of growing up, our path to adulthood often referred to as a rite of passage.

One of the biggest concerns I had, starting before I was even a teen, was when I would be considered a woman. I wanted to know what that meant, who was one and who wasn't, when I'd get to be one, and if being a woman related to a particular age or something more ethereal, as I suspected it did.

When I was thirteen, I turned to my dad and told him I wanted people to refer to me as a woman. I was sick and tired of being one of "the girls," as my sister and I were constantly referred to. I was tired of being thought of as less capable or less important than the other adults I lived with. I felt like my opinions were thought of as less important and I wanted to be treated equally.

I actually had it pretty good, come to think of it. My dad clearly intended for Sophia and me to live and function with the rest of the adults we shared a home and a life with as much as possible. I got to sit in on the frequent house meetings when everyone took turns talking about their daily lives and anything that was on their mind. When doing group projects or making changes to the house, I was welcome to share my opinion on how I thought things should be done. Sophia and I even formed our own businesses throughout our childhood and were given free rein to form and execute our business plans.

By thirteen, I was treated in a quite adult-like way, but it wasn't enough. I was done with being considered a "little girl." I had a period, I had boobs, and I was physically strong enough to whup just about anyone I cared to (I was after all a boxer and soccer player). My dad turned to me as we walked down our dirt driveway, side by side, and told me that when I was a woman, I wouldn't have to ask people to call me one.

I can still feel the dark flush that rushed down my body when he said that. I knew the truth of it, even if it wasn't the answer I'd been looking for. I figured that if I asked people to think of me in a particular way, they'd do it. It seemed pretty simple.

Now that I'm closer to thirty than I am twenty, I am beginning to consistently think of myself as a woman. Sometimes in my head, I'm still a little kid. I feel the frustration of small problems, or the weight of my responsibilities that I'd much rather shrug off. Or I take pleasure in uncomplicated things, like ladybugs walking along a log. Or approving of another person just because they are there, free of my expectations. And even though I've been noodling over my personal concept of the term "woman" for quite some time, my definition is still in flux. Growing up is a process and it looks different for everyone. Whether they subscribe to "woman" or "man" or "girl" or "boy" or "they/them" or another label altogether, each person's experience of transitioning from childhood to adulthood is completely unique and worth celebrating for its own personal individuality.

I happened to come into solo Internet usage at the same time the social media website Myspace was rising in popularity. Before then, the main thing I'd do on a computer was research for the essays I was learning to write in my homeschool English Comp classes and chat with my cousins and nephews in Ohio through AIM (the now-defunct messaging application by AOL). We'd met once or twice before but having access to a computer on which we could instantly chat with them and thus build relationships quickly and from afar was terribly exciting for my sister and me. We began spending increasingly long stints of time on the family computer and it was through those relatives that we first heard about Myspace. Quickly, we built profiles and found more and more people that we knew on the site—from our relatives all the way across the country to our soccer teammates that we saw nearly every day.

For the first time, social media became a presence in our lives. When I was fifteen I went to the piercing parlor in Ashland to have my first cartilage piercing—a small hoop placed on the upper portion of my right ear. Back home a few days later, I contorted my body into the classic "Myspace Pose": slightly sideways, pointing the camera at yourself from above, and looking up at the camera with a slight head-cock. This time, I flaunted a new piercing. Plugging my point-and-shoot camera into my computer, I extracted the best picture and layered a few filters over it until I had the same picture but in high-contrast red and orange tones. Posting that picture, and the onslaught of approval that followed, made the piercing "Myspace Official."

All this talk about Myspace and point-and-shoot cameras is dating me, but I'm confident that you could replace any of these descriptions of Myspace with

Facebook or Snapchat or Instagram or whatever's popular these days and get a pretty clear picture of what I'm talking about. This was the beginning of being able to see into other people's lives without their knowledge and the ability to present an online version of yourself to strangers as well as friends that you had near total control of.

There was one phenomenon particular to Myspace where users could post various forms of surveys or lists, usually consisting of things you have or have not done. A "Things I've Done" bulletin was usually a long list with about thirty or forty activities, and you'd check or uncheck the ones you had or had not done. Like: held hands, had a buzz cut, your hair is longer than your bf/gf, performed oral sex, received oral sex, left the country, and on and on.

As I said, these things were really popular. You got to see your friends' responses and then fill the same form out yourself and sort of compare where you were at. I adored filling them out. In fact, I had to limit myself from doing each one that came up for fear I'd be deemed an excessive weirdo for spending my time filling out pointless Myspace Notes, so a couple a week were all I would allow myself.

It was a way of showing off what you'd done, what you hadn't done (but might like to), and seeing where you sized up in relation to the "norm" (one's pool of Myspace contacts seemed like a fair representation of the rest of the world at the time).

Everyone wants to know how they are doing in comparison to the "norm." Even people who say they don't, do in some area of their life. This is an extremely common concern when it comes to sensuality in general and can be a great inhibitor. Instead of reaching for what we want individually, we look to see what those around us (or on our social media platforms) have and may base our choices off of what we see.

· · · · · ·

Before this chapter concludes, I have one more thing to say about growing up and rites of passage.

• • • • • •

There is one typical rite of passage that I find to be quite outdated, even though it continues to survive in our modern society: virginity. Mainly, that it exists. Or that it's a valid way of viewing and judging other humans (virgins and non-virgins) or deciding on a potential partner (are they a virgin?). In an age where we carry technology advanced enough to send another human to space and where multitudes of people are experiencing the freedom (and, even more novel: the safety) to express their gender in ways other than the one assigned at birth, surely we can let go of this putrid notion of virginity.

For those unaware, a "virgin" is someone who has not experienced penis-vagina sex before. In the past, a woman's worth was tied to whether or not she was a virgin. Much of this had to do with religion and, to put it frankly, money. Marriageability (and thus the potential bride-price) hinged on her sexual history.

This is problematic for a number of reasons. From a sensualist's perspective, this is a pain-oriented conundrum. The myth of virginity essentially communicates that the worth of a woman diminishes once she's been penetrated by a man. In actuality, nothing changes. Absolutely nothing. The first time I put a penis inside of me, I was unchanged immediately after, the next morning, and in the years to follow. How you feel about yourself, your partner, or about sex as a whole may shift, but that's up to you.

From a larger point of view, it's an unequal playing field for men and women since the man's value does not change after having intercourse with a woman. In fact, if anything, he actually becomes more valuable because now he's "experienced" and thus more attractive. Young men are encouraged to go "sow their wild oats" and basically have all the sex they want because, you know, "boys will be boys" and it's part of their rite of passage; it's part of growing up.

And to make this perspective a bit bigger, it's a severely limiting perspective on human sexuality that only focuses on heterosexual (female-male) sex. What about men that have sex with men? Or women with women? Or gender non-conforming with others? Or asexuality, for that matter? Are they all to remain virgins if they never have P-V sex? On one hand, it's a bit of an exclusion that perhaps serves a nicer purpose; that is, non-traditional sexuality doesn't have to subscribe to a cultural bag of rocks that millions of people have dealt with. And on the other hand, perhaps that's a signal that times have changed and it's time to rework our collective narrative around sexuality.

• • • • • •

Let's lose the loss of virginity. It's time for a new term to describe our early sexual experiences, creating pleasure-focused labels for our experiences that, instead of focusing on loss, focus on what we gain, or the benefits of the experience. It has been suggested that perhaps a new, improved definition of virginity could be when a person has their first orgasm with another person.[11] When I first came across this notion, in an NPR interview with Peggy Orenstein, author of *Girls & Sex*,[12] I was simultaneously floored and then inspired to take this definition on for myself.

Growing up in a community surrounded by winning viewpoints on sensuality and a whole force of encouraging friends who only wanted me to have positive experiences during my foray into sexual activity, I fell into this trap myself.

When I wanted to have intercourse with a man for the first time, I went about the experience deliberately. I talked it over with my friends, I talked it over with the guy I wanted to do it with, who is also one of my closest friends, I gave myself time and space to consider if it was what I actually wanted, and then when I decided that I was in fact "ready," I planned the time and place of the event.

The act itself was a lot of fun and is a memory that I treasure. I took the time to light a few candles before we did it, because I figured, why the heck not. Looking back on that evening in bed together, I see green walls lit with soft light, I remember the feel of my velvet nighty against my skin. I remember laughter and talking. We had a few peaks and eventually I decided that I'd had enough so we stopped. I felt happy afterwards and had that sensation of being wrapped up in something new. That was the first time I'd had another person inside of me in that particular way and it was somewhat alien. Surprisingly odd and foreign, despite my various mock-ups and imaginings.

And afterwards, I still managed to describe the experience as "losing my virginity." Where was the loss? With retrospect, it was an addition. It was the first act of many to come and was simply a new experience that I'd decided to have. Nothing was taken away from me or physically altered.

· · · · · ·

Before I had intercourse for the first time, I thought of it as a rite of passage amongst many. First period, first kiss, first intercourse, as well as boobs and hairs of course. All of these are hallmarks along the journey we call "adulthood." This path looks different for everyone depending on culture, sexual orientation, gender identity, and a myriad of factors. Not experiencing a standard cultural rite of passage does not make a person less than or even different. As an adult, I have realized how much pressure I've placed on myself in the past to achieve certain hallmarks or achievements that our society has deemed "good." There are so many hurdles as we grow and age that eventually we realize that some of us choose certain experiences, while others choose another: it's your choice and is entirely up to you as to when and if you'd like to experience a particular rite of passage.

However, from a pleasure-oriented perspective, we can begin to view ourselves and our sensuality differently, without the standard pressures of our culture and without the need to compare ourselves to "the norm." In the following chapters, I will describe aspects of sensuality and human sexuality with a pleasure-oriented lens and introduce a new framing for forms of self-care, friendship and relationship building, and sex itself.

Chapter 4

MENARCHE AND HEAT CYCLES (WE REALLY ARE MAMMALS, AFTER ALL)

When I first heard about periods, I immediately wanted one. I hopped off the bed that my sister and I had both been seated on for our first Female Body class that my mom taught and made a beeline for the bathroom. Perched on the toilet seat while I relieved myself, I gave a few extra pushes to get things moving inside, and then, after wiping, I peered down at my soiled tissue paper, fully expecting to see blood and for my first period to have officially begun.

Of course, I was slightly disappointed when what I saw looked the same as it always did. In fact, it'd be another four years until I actually experienced menarche, to use the official term for a person's first menstruation. I would spend the next four years eagerly anticipating this event which became, in my mind, the first official step I'd make toward full-blown womanhood. Since I lived in a house full of women, I utilized them to extract every tidbit of information about periods that I could. On my daily training runs around the hilly dirt roads of our property, I'd query my running partners about when they'd gotten their first period, what a period felt like, and what kind of products they used to handle the situation. I didn't limit myself to soley the women I lived with, as I was known for cornering various visitors and taking advantage of their polite friendliness to acquire more data about this elusive monthly visitor. A seemingly innocuous summertime visit to our swimming hole was likely to turn into a lengthy discussion about the hows and whys of menstruation and anything else about puberty that I could draw out of them. No subject was too precious, nothing was sacred, and modesty was simply not a notion I was acquainted with.

Having a sister who was a year older than me allowed for a preview of the changes to come. Of course, she got everything first: armpit hairs, leg hairs, breasts, the list goes on. You name it, she got it first. However, just because we were sisters didn't mean it was a free-for-all in the information department. In fact, she was quite secretive. I'll never forget the afternoon that I surprised her in the bathroom as she opened the shower door to reach for a dry towel after her shower. The steam parted to reveal my sister, fully naked except for a large wet washcloth plastered to the front of her body. Where I expected to find boobs and hairy parts, I instead found a washcloth and face that read simultaneous embarrassment and outrage.

My sister wasn't such a fan of the changes she was going through. I knew she had a period when I started seeing pink plastic wrapped pads pilling up next to her dresser in our shared bedroom. Her preference for baggy T-shirts and pants made it nearly impossible to detect the stages of breast development that I knew must be occurring, according to pencil-drawing illustrations I was obsessing over from our Female Body class. We no longer waltzed around our bedroom naked together, and instead she made an effort to hide her body at all times.

Years later, now that her breasts are fully developed of course, we have talked extensively about our experiences of puberty and she's clued me in on how private she felt about that time in her life. It wasn't easy for her; she has told me how she wished that she could put the brakes on her development in any way she could. Unable to do so, she hid what was happening and hated what she saw in the mirror. Eventually, she changed her mind and did a complete one-eighty and opened her arms (and neckline) to her transition from girlhood to womanhood. And now, she's one of the most confident, body-positive people that I know, and at times reminds me to stop being hard on myself or to stop viewing my body negatively. Go figure.

Needless to say, she got her period before I did. I figured it was inevitable that she would; she was a grade ahead of me in our homeschool classes, her boobs were bigger than mine (I could detect this from furtive glances her way when I knew she was changing clothes), and she was managing to stay a full five inches ahead of me in height, so why wouldn't she get her period before me? Ours being the kind of family that it is, all of the women in our community threw her a First

Period Party to celebrate her maturation. I, however, was not invited and it was one of the few parties that my sister attended that I wasn't there for. Lingering outside the closed door of their Period Party, the laughter that drifted out into the hallway stung me to my core. Three years of anxiously awaiting my own period came down to this, an official party that all my friends got to go to but me.

Noticing me, my dad called over to me from his spot on the couch in our living room. Cuddled on the leather sofa, we watched the winter Olympics together. The sweetness of that evening with my Dad, partners in our lack of periods, is something I recall just as vividly as my own Period Party a year later.

I did eventually get a period. But not before my childhood best friend, who was a year younger than me, got hers. Each time I compared myself to my peers, I felt worse and my self-appointed pressure continued to mount. Pressure to grow, pressure to change, pressure to achieve these set steps of womanhood. Granted, that wasn't always my reality; there were days I'd forget periods were even a thing. Or better yet, I'd remember that once I got a period, I wouldn't *not* have one for what seemed like forever, so I'd better just enjoy what's happening right now. At age eleven, the prospect of menopause seemed impossibly distant, just as the mere six days of anticipation between soccer games seemed to take eons.

It must have been early spring, because we were out in the garden tilling the plots with the aid of our backhoe. The dirt was dark and cold, and I recall the heavy feeling of hard work in my body, the dirt drying and cracking on the skin of my hands, the cool sweat on my brow. The gray, richly overcast sky contrasted the heavy earth that our whole family worked together.

I walked inside to pee, somewhat dreading the activity because it meant so many steps: removing my mud-caked boots, washing my dirt-covered hands, and peeling down my dusty pants, all for a short bit of relief when I could've just gone in the garden and skipped all this tedium. As I shoved down my jeans I saw it. Thick, rusty brown blood on my blue paisley underwear. My first thought was a question—"what the hell is that?" But, of course, I knew. It had finally happened. The day had come.

I walked out of that bathroom and felt like I was floating. My first plan was to keep this news to myself, as Sophia had done. And in a family so prone to open communication and discussing everything directly, I finally had an actual secret that seemed worth holding on to. This was something that occurred in *my* body and was all mine to know and feel and experience. It had nothing to do with anyone but me.

But, that plan lasted for about five seconds longer than it took me to think it. I'm not one to keep a story like that to myself (as you can see). I found my mom and gave her the news and that information quickly spread throughout our community. Another party was planned, and this time, I was in. My sister and I sat together on a couch surrounded by the women in our life, our mothers, and we laughed and told stories together. Fifteen years later, I can still see around that room and watch big, open smiles and the bright lights of happy women. It was a beautiful introduction to womanhood; a welcoming to the circle.

I've had approximately two hundred periods since and while some of the novelty has worn off since then, it's still there. Each month my menstruation is something I anticipate and recognize as an ongoing cycle within my body. I experience a difference in the energy I feel in my body before, during, and after menstruating as well as during ovulation. It's a cycle that plays a role in each day of my life. I was raised to value my period as a beautiful aspect of being a woman, something to welcome. I think a lot of that early obsession was partially because it seemed like something fun; it was an experience I knew my friends related over and I wanted to be part of the conversation. Of course, I knew it wasn't all rainbows and butterflies. I knew cramps would hurt and believe me they do. And bloating, breast tenderness, lethargy, mood shifts; none of that is something to laugh at. But instead of viewing this negatively, or as a "syndrome," I was offered the viewpoint that it's an experience and that I can have it positively just the way it is.

As it turns out, most people don't get to experience their periods that way. Apparently, it's something that there's a lot of stigma attached to. Well, that's why this book had to be written and why I'm glad you're reading it. Over half of the world's population has had a period at some point in their lives and every human being on this earth came from someone who had a period. So, it's something to be grateful for: it's a natural part of being a human and having a uterus. The negative social stigma is totally unnecessary.

• • • • • •

When a person is on their period they're never just simply on their period. The company Clue (a period-tracking app company) recently conducted a global study which found that there are over five thousand slang terms for menstruation. Examples of slang terms for menstruation are being "on the rag," it's "shark week," or it's "that time of the month."[1] Most of these terms do not have positive connotations and don't accurately describe what's going on. Using veiled language, or language that is inherently negative, prohibits conversation and leads to greater mystery.[2]

There are plenty of taboos about menstruation, some of which is cultural and some of which is based in pure misinformation. Menstrual taboos are referred to in the Bible, Quran, and even the earliest Latin encyclopedia.[3] This negativity is rampant and socially acceptable. The time leading up to and during menstruation has been medically labeled as "PMS" or premenstrual syndrome. By calling it a "syndrome" we attach an unnecessarily negative connotation to menstruation. Some women do experience intense, even extreme, amounts of cramps, bleeding, and other experiences as part of their periods, which can have a debilitating impact on their daily life. However, that has been medically redefined as PMDD (Premenstrual Dysphoric Disorder) which approximately 3 to 8 percent of people who have periods experience.[4] The other common experiences that some women experience during periods have been redefined as "symptoms" as opposed to a "syndrome." When people refer to "PMS" they usually mean experiences like mood swings, headaches, cramps, and a myriad of other symptoms which are rarely debilitating. Popular culture and our media have not, however, learned to distinguish these nuances and still report that the majority of women experience extreme PMS and promote the idea that medical assistance is required for people with periods.

Psychologist Robyn Stein DeLuca has researched this topic extensively and spoke about it publicly in her TEDx talk "The Good News about PMS." In her work, she points out the effects that these negative messages have on people with periods. Research has shown that when the message is communicated that all people with periods experience PMS, a person is more likely to think that, they too, experience it even when their actual reported experiences of their periods do not indicate PMS. DeLuca also argues that the widespread myth of PMS serves to invalidate women's emotions, pointing out that "when people respond to a woman's anger with the thought, 'Oh, it's just that time of the month,' her ability to be taken seriously or effect change is severely limited."[5]

Too often a woman is told she is "PMSing" when she's just being forthright, standing up for herself, or speaking up. And, it ultimately becomes a way to discredit and discount women. If she's acting a particular way (from flakey to angry to bossy; it varies widely) she may be labeled as having PMS, regardless of where she's at in her cycle. Eye-rolls and agreement will surely follow, and whatever she was doing will be ignored. A recent public example of this was in the 2008 presidential primary when Hillary Clinton was frequently referred to as being unfit for the presidency due to "PMS and the mood swings."[6] The name-calling that comes along with being a person who menstruates is just one example of the negative conditioning layered on these basic aspects of being human. Ultimately, it's sexism and you don't have to buy it.

And actually, in my personal experience, periods can be fun. What is actually happening is an increase in energy, which can be interpreted negatively or positively. Sometimes I use this increase in energy to be more creative. I'll feel inspired to write more or to complete projects that have been on my list for a while. Or sometimes my cramps will be particularly intense and all I can do is take a bath and then a nap. While I experience a range from month to month, overall, it's a time when I become more aware of my body. There are many changes happening all the time; sometimes I feel heavy, sometimes I feel like my skin is buzzing. The sensation in my body can change from moment to moment. I also become more aware of my own anatomy: sometimes my cramps are incredibly revealing regarding the exact location of my uterus or my ovaries. I like seeing what my body produces and having attention on what my body can do.

By being aware of your body and noticing what you feel, you can make the right choice for yourself and you don't have to go into the experience perceiving it negatively.

What It Is

So what is menstruation, exactly? Menstruation is the monthly bleeding when bodies with uteri shed the uterine lining, which is called the *endometrium*. Menstrual fluid flows from the uterus, sometimes referred to as the "womb," through the small opening in the cervix and passes out of the body through the vagina. Menstruation happens if the egg that the ovaries release during ovulation isn't fertilized by sperm. This causes hormone levels to drop, which then causes the lining inside the uterus to shed, as the lining is no longer required as it would be for a fertilized egg (also called an *ovum*). The lining of the uterus would have become the placenta if the ovum had been fertilized.[7]

The average menstrual cycle is twenty-eight days long, from the first day you start bleeding to the start of your next period. The first day of bleeding is marked as the first day of your period and menstrual cycle, as it is the most obvious sign in the entire cycle. The start of bleeding is the most reliable marker because some people experience a lot of spotting at the end of their periods, which makes the last day of a period difficult to determine, and because ovulation is virtually hidden and can be difficult to track. Cycles can range anywhere from twenty-one to thirty-five days in adults and from twenty-five to forty-five days in young teens. Most periods, which is when the actual bleeding occurs, last from three to five days. Biologically, the body is preparing for pregnancy in the weeks before bleeding starts.[8]

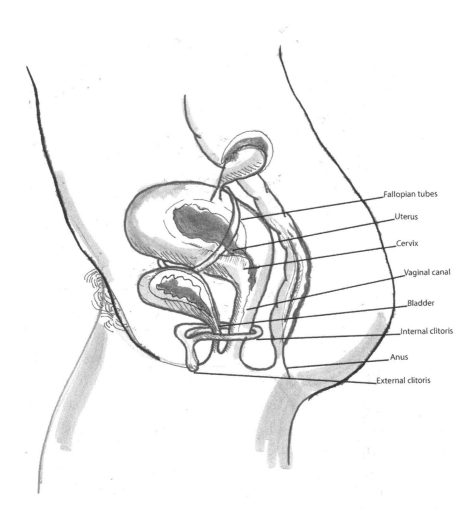

Fallopian tubes

Uterus

Cervix

Vaginal canal

Bladder

Internal clitoris

Anus

External clitoris

In this image you can see some of the major players in the female reproductive system: the uterus (where a fetus can grow), ovaries (which stores and releases the ova/egg and also produces hormones), which are connected to fallopian tubes which is what the ova travel through to the uterus. The cervix is located at the end of the vaginal canal and serves as the opening to the uterus. The cervix has a tiny opening called the *os* which is mostly closed but can dilate. The vaginal canal is partly wrapped by that wonderful internal part of the clitoris which we spoke so highly of earlier in this book, when engorged. For the most part, the vaginal canal is in a collapsed state but since it is both flexible and muscular, it can expand to accommodate whatever is put inside. Contrary to popular belief, the vaginal canal is actually curved upward toward the cervix, not straight.[9]

During the menstrual cycle, if fertilization does not occur, the lining which has been prepared in the uterus sheds and leaves the body through the cervix by way of the vaginal canal. The menstrual cycle actually begins in the brain with the release of certain substances which stimulate the pituitary gland which then releases two hormones: follicle-stimulating hormone (FSH) and luteinizing hormone (LH). This sets off a series of changes in the fallopian tubes which have an egg develop. If this egg is not fertilized with sperm then your progesterone (the hormone which was getting a lot of these balls rolling) will drop, which will cause your period to begin.[10]

Menstruation isn't just your period, either. It's part of a month-long (typically a twenty-one to thirty-one day) cycle that occurs in your body when you have a uterus and female reproductive parts. It's comprised of three parts: menstruation, proliferative phase (building of the endometrium and preparing for fertilization), and the secretory or luteal phase (when the egg is released and ready to be fertilized). During each part of the cycle, different changes and hormonal shifts occur. While we mainly talk about the menstrual or period part of the cycle, each day brings a different change and is a different part of the whole cycle.[11]

Unlike males, females are born with all of the eggs (or ova) that they will have in their lifetime. Females start off with about one to two million and will end up releasing around five hundred.[12] Males continually produce sperm starting in puberty through the remainder of their life.[13]

In a short break from our regularly scheduled menstruation programming, we're going to discuss male reproductive anatomy.

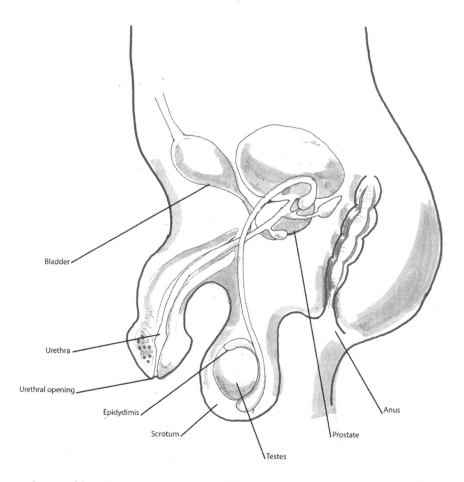

Bladder

Urethra

Urethral opening

Epidydimis

Scrotum

Testes

Prostate

Anus

Pictured here is a representation of the testes, (also called testicles or balls) which is where hormones and the sperm cells are produced. The testes (of which there are typically two) are divided by a thin wall of tissue and covered by a sac of skin and muscle called the scrotum. The testes connect through a series of organs and tubes (namely the epididymis and spermatic cord) which leads to the penis through the urethra and exits the penis through the urethral opening. The urethra is a small tube (roughly eight inches long) which connects the bladder, testes, and the ejaculatory ducts. Fluid exits the penis through the urethra. In this drawing you can also see the prostate, a small very sensitive gland which wraps around part of the urethra and is located in the canal between the rectum and anus. Another important part of this anatomy is the erectile tissue, the two corpora cavernosa and the corpus spongiosum, which are the three long cylinders that run the length of the penis and engorge with blood when erect. Erection is caused by blood filling these areas during arousal. Erections are possible from the very beginning of life[14] although the ability to ejaculate arrives after puberty starts. Which does not mean the ability to experience orgasm only happens in puberty, as orgasm can (and does) happen without ejaculation.[15]

• • • • • •

Back to periods.

The average age for menarche (first period) in the United States is twelve. But, that can vary wildly: menarche can happen anytime between the ages of eight and fifteen. It can take several years for your period to become "regular," that is, approximately twenty-eight days long with two to three days of deviation. After menarche, you may skip periods or have wildly varying lengths to your cycle, which is perfectly normal.[16]

Later on in life comes menopause. This is when a woman stops having periods; it's a transitional period that can last two to eight years. After this transition, she stops producing eggs and can no longer get pregnant. There are many hormonal shifts that occur during this time. As with menstruation, menopause is a heavily stigmatized life-transition that, again, all people with uteri experience.[17]

There is one more myth to bust before we change topics: period blood isn't really that bloody. Menstruation is the shedding of your uterine lining, vaginal cells, discharge, and some blood. Flow can vary from person to person, and it averages at about six to twelve teaspoons overall. Every woman's flow is different, and it can vary from cycle to cycle. Your "heavy" may be another person's "medium" or even "light." There is a wide range.[18]

Period Care

Self-care is key when it comes to your period, and the concept of "self-care" looks different for different people. As I mentioned earlier, menstruation is just one part of an ongoing cycle. By being aware of where you are in your cycle, you can prepare for and begin to anticipate your period. Eating well, drinking lots of water, and getting enough rest will have your period experience feel better. I highly recommend exercise as a way to ease your menstrual experience, even if it's just a daily walk.[19]

There are many options when it comes to taking care of the monthly visit. My grandma and my mom's generations (and the women who came before them) had fewer options to take care of their periods than people do now. Long before adhesive pads were invented, the "sanitary belt" was available, which essentially worked like a garter belt for a thick, long, absorbent pad.[20] Now there are pads available in all shapes, sizes, and absorbencies, as well as tampons, reusable menstrual cups, and assorted other methods. And since the US Food and Drug Administration approved the first hormonal birth control (usually referred to as "the pill") in 1960,[21] many people do not regularly experience periods, as some oral contraceptives prevent periods from occurring.[22]

But if you do get a period, there are entire companies and apps dedicated to selling products to make it a safer, cleaner, more convenient experience for you. Some tampon companies will deliver monthly packages containing tampons that have been personalized for you depending on the intensity and duration of your period. In order to provide a more "green" period, companies are also creating tampons and pads that are made with natural and safer materials. Bleach-free and compostable products are readily available.[23]

Also rising in popularity are reusable products. There are many varieties on the market, including menstrual cups (silicone cups which are inserted into the vagina and emptied throughout the day), reusable pads (made of absorbent material), and menstrual underwear which absorb your flow. I highly recommend finding a reusable product that works for you. When I first started my period, I mainly used pads and only used tampons when a situation required it, like swimming. As I became more familiar with my period and handling the fluid each month, I became curious about branching out and finding products that actually worked for me and fit my lifestyle better. Eventually I landed on a completely reusable system (a menstrual cup and reusable pads) which cuts down on my monthly costs as well as reduces my environmental impact.

In conclusion, suffice it to say that menstruation is a common coming of age marker in girls' lives. If you've got a uterus, you're most likely going to learn about periods, whether you want to or not. If you were provided a sex ed class in school, they covered menstruation. If your parents or guardian talked to you about puberty, they probably covered periods. If you happened to pick up some other book on puberty, they, too, covered that time of the month. Sex ed tends to focus on topics having to do with the mechanics of your body and your safety. So, I probably haven't told you much you didn't already know.

Too often the conversations end there. We find out we are able to get pregnant and why, but what does it feel like? What about the stuff besides bleeding? What about pleasure?

As I've stressed earlier in this book, I'm big on the experiential aspects of life. It's good to know the mechanical aspects of what's going on, whether that's something in your body, because often that leads to a better understanding of how we move and feel through the world. But the tendency is to rely on scientific explanations and rarely discuss the felt and unseen aspects of our experience. And thus, we handicap ourselves. What do you do with the parts if you don't know how to read the manual? In this chapter we discussed what a period is and how to handle it, but we haven't delved into much of the experience. In this next section, I will discuss some of the more experiential aspects of menstruation as well as other cycles that are at play simultaneously.

Heat Cycles

Sophia and I would play a game as we laid in bed at night, before our parents came to tuck us in. Saying "goodnight" to each other was a nightly ritual that, if skipped, could cause great emotional turmoil on our end. At times when we'd be separated by travel or circumstance, and if we were unable to get a call through due to bad timing or any number of obstacles, tears were sure to be shed.

But this particular evening, we were all under the same roof. Sophia and I, wrapped up in our dark room and ensconced in sheets, blankets, and pillows, were far from sleepy. We chatted away about our day, the people in our lives, and any number of important topics. Energy moved through our bodies like bright headlights shooting by on a freeway at night. Blurs following blurs and we talked more and more, our energy escalating in peaks, alternating between a new topic and assuring each other that it was time to go to sleep.

Upon realizing our parents *still* hadn't come in, a slight sense of worry began to bubble. Were they already in bed? Had they forgotten? Shutting up for a moment, we listened together and sure enough, we could hear the halting symphonics of voices rising and falling in the living room. Clearly, they were still up and at it, which only left the latter as a possibility. Adding to this, we'd already been in bed for quite some time, long enough to exhaust our various matters of discussion and pick up this new game, at the very least.

Being forgotten brewed and bubbled to a point of real concern, which only made us want them to come in for a goodnight visit all the more. We decided to will them to us. Closing our eyes and focusing intensely on our parents, we thought as hard as we could about them coming in our room. We figured we could simply pull them into the room with our thoughts if we wanted it badly enough. Laying there, silent but burning with a particular heat in our bodies, we willed them, each in our own way. A few minutes later, a sliver of light filled the entryway as a door cracked open and our dad poked his head in. We reveled; joyous in equal parts at his appearance and our accomplishment. Thrilled, I told him what we'd been doing, that we willed him into our room. I expected surprise, or even confusion at what I'd told him, but I received none of that. His reaction was one of "of course," as he'd known he'd come to the door for a reason.

There is a way that we feel and respond to each other throughout our daily lives that few want to discuss. It's an undercurrent, a web of sensations akin to a human system of mycorrhiza, through which we silently communicate. Perhaps another sense to add to our growing list. This ability to feel and be felt has not diminished as I've grown. I even learned on an intellectual level how we call and respond to one another as any other mammal does in our great animal kingdom. Having these words said aloud, I of course understood them, but I'd often argue or begin to wonder about how it actually worked.

The concept of how people feel and respond to each other probably sounds pretty woo-woo but bear with me. The remainder of this chapter is largely based on my personal experience of living in a group surrounded by self-appointed sensual researchers, that is, people who had deliberately chosen a life where they acknowledged their own perceptions and how they experienced other people and told the truth about all of it. Not only is this how we function together, but this mode of relating was given just as much weight as the scientifically-backed, peer-reviewed facts that sometimes supported the viewpoints from which we operated, and sometimes did not. This is all to say that much of what is to follow does *not* have support from our scientific or medical communities simply because there is very little research available concerning heat cycles in humans. So skip ahead to the next chapter if you're not interested in my personal theories about how our bodies function together.

• • • • • •

As I alluded to earlier, a menstrual cycle is one of many cycles in a woman's body. We are mammals, after all, and mammals respond to various amounts of energy available throughout the year, in situations, and on the individual level. Each month, just as the moon transitions through its cycle of waxing and waning, so does a woman's body. This cycle is also called a "lunar cycle" for that very reason. Within each month, varying levels of energy are available. Five days to a week before menstruation begins, the most amount of energy is available in a woman's body. There is also a spike during ovulation, for obvious reproductive reasons.

This increase in energy takes a lot of forms. It's been heavily medicalized in our society and, as explored earlier in this chapter, the tag "PMS" (Premenstrual Syndrome) is often used. By labeling it a "syndrome" we unnecessarily associate this time in a woman's life as being painful. But really, it's an increase in energy.

I've noticed a few signs that come along when someone is about to menstruate. These can be dilated pupils, darkening of color around eyes (often called a "pregnancy mask"), craving gooey or salty foods, and a change in body odor. Irritability and bitchiness sometimes come with this change; as a woman experiences this increase of energy close to the start of her period, how she chooses to use it can vary. These signs may or may not be present in every woman, as each person's experience is unique.

As her cycle progresses toward menstruation, more and more energy is available. Her body fills with this energy, closer and closer until the "release" of menstruation, which can feel like letting air out of a balloon. These signs are not exclusive to those five to seven days before a period begins; it could be, or it could be another heat cycle at play. There are different cycles happening from birth to death. Women are born with this capacity for energy and it remains with us until our last days, regardless of whether or not we're menstruating.

Since we're mammals, there are no heat cycles in males. In the mammalian world, the female, not the male, goes into heat. The male's response is correlated to females in heat.[24]

Depending on where you live, you may be able to poke your head out your door and see it all around you. I grew up in a rural area and we've always raised a variety of animals. Goats are a great example of the heat cycle phenomenon. Our billy goat is huge, hairy, and odorous. Most of the time he's by himself and he's happy; as long as he has enough hay to munch on he's pretty reasonable. The does are kept nearby but are separate from him for most of the time and each little group goes about the business of their lives in relative peace and quiet. That is until the does go into heat. Suddenly, the billy becomes a raging maniac trying to get at them. He yells, he stomps, he stretches across the dividing fence, as if nearness would satisfy the burning, raging yearning inside of him. The does are noticeably more interested in him, too. Prancing back and forth, they waft their pheromones and continue putting out the call. Once they're out of heat things go back to normal.

Periods are just one of four cycles that are at play. We are warm-blooded animals, which means we respond to changes in the temperature as the earth makes it's 365-day journey around the sun. As you're well aware, we've divided the year up into four different seasons which correlate to our proximity on the earth to the sun. I live in North America and the following seasonal changes are specific to the northern hemisphere. In the southern hemisphere, the cycle is flipped.

The lowest energy season of the *annual cycle* is winter. Frankly, it's cold. There is less sunlight available, the days are shorter, and the nights are longer. You can see that it's a low-energy time in a myriad of ways: animals are hibernating, the deciduous trees have died back, and there is very little plant growth.

When I think of winter from when I was growing up, I imagine the dark, bare oaks that surrounded our property. Their long, scraggly branches seemed to reach up to the sky, naked, except for the large clumps of mistletoe that were always clinging. That particular plant seemed like the only thing around with any aggression left in it, everything else felt quiet and still. There is a particular steely, icy feel that the air gets to it, so that any time I leave the house I'm immediately reminded that winter is here. This is a slow time of year.

Springtime has the highest energy in the annual cycle. This is where the whole idea of "spring fever" derives. There is an abundance of energy available, and we go from the lowest amount to the highest amount available in a yearly cycle. The *Encyclopædia Britannica* describes this response in terms of the increase in light available: "Light, usually in the form of increasing day length, seems to be the major environmental stimulus for most vertebrates [. . .] That this should be such an important factor is quite reasonable in an evolutionary sense: increasing day length signifies the onset of a favorable period for reproduction."[25] That jump from winter to spring can feel like a virtual springboard. Suddenly, the quiet, sluggishness of winter gives way to growth and emergence. There is more light available as we progress toward the longest day of the year and more light has a dramatic effect on the flora and fauna. In agrarian societies, this is when the planting happens and when we lay the groundwork of the harvest for the rest of the year.

From spring, we transition to summer which is the second lowest amount of energy in the yearly cycle. Summer is when you watch the crops grow and activities are more laid-back. School is out, and the days lack the busy bluster of spring. The fall is the second highest amount of energy; it's a fun peak before winter slips in again. This is when the harvest occurs and there is a lot going on—football season begins, and school is back in session. The vibrant colors of fall begin to darken and shift toward the cooling and closing down of winter time.

Besides the annual cycle, we also have *situational cycles*. This is when women are affected by other women. One result of this can be menstrual cycles aligning. There has been scientific research on this topic since the 1970s, but results are inconclusive and heavily debated.[26] Personally, I experience situational heat cycles in a way that is more complex than my period arriving later or earlier than usual.

I grew up with a lot of women and looking back, "situational heat cycle" is a dry term to describe some of the warmest and sweetest times in my life. Visions of beautiful women in pretty clothes grouped around the kitchen talking and laughing—that kind of laughter that builds and crescendos in a big wave of uproar that washes over everyone in the room. Or the moments of sitting around the living room, when an idea sparks and spreads across my friends, lighting up each one individually and the room as a whole. Ideas begin to pile up, one on top of the other until everyone in the room is filled up and inspired to begin. Situational heat cycles are women feeling each other and noticing one another. In my experience, women who live together or work together tend to go into heat together.

Women can also turn on all by themselves, for no other reason than wanting to do so.[27] This is pretty uncommon in the animal kingdom; in fact, there only a few animals like dolphins and bonobos that have volitional heat. Most mammals go into heat seasonally, like our goats going into heat in the spring and fall.[28]

Turn on, volitional heat, is closely linked to approval. When I'm approving and in agreement, I'm turned on. My turn on can be focused on a particular person; it can be broad; and it can even be about an activity or inanimate object. For me, turn on is a warm glow. It's being happy with how things are. It's feeling good and letting people know. Sometimes I look at a particular person and send those good feelings right to them. Every once in a while, it will be acknowledged with a smile, but most of the time it passes unmarked. Sometimes it's feeling pleased with a project.

While some do not have heat cycles themselves, they can notice the heat cycles in women. It is common for people, both men and women, to judge women for their energy. Women are constantly dismissed for "PMS" or "being on the rag," as if a woman is somehow incapacitated by this part of her life. Instead of passing judgment, you can notice and pay attention to the people in your life during all of these cycles.

These cycles can be fun to watch and experience if you are paying attention. Charting your cycle is one way to do this. There are modern conveniences like Clue or other period tracking apps. Charting a cycle keeps you aware of what is going on in your, or a female in your life's, body.

How women experience all of these cycles can vary widely. With the monthly cycle, some women's periods pass without a thought and some have very intense cycles that they manage with birth control, or other medical options.

Across the board, when a woman decides to experience her life pleasurably, it has an effect on her physical experience. Through learning about cycles and the different amounts of energy available throughout the year, month, and day, a woman can become more aware. Once you are more aware, you can make pleasurable choices from that place. One of the most effective ways to add pleasure into your life is through self-care and, in particular, through masturbation, but more on that in the next chapter.

Part 2
Sex and Sensuality

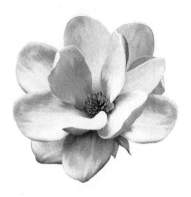

Chapter 5

"THE M-THING" AND TAKING CARE OF YOUR BODY

When I was seven, I couldn't find my clitoris. I learned at some point that I had one; I probably found out about it during a pre-pubescent Female Body Class or in some precursor mother-daughter conversation. I had heard that it was a small "bump" of sorts near the top of my genitals that contained a lot of nerve endings, or something to that effect. I know that I thought the clitoris was *very* important and I felt that I should definitely know where it was, so I felt a bit of pressure to find this thing. Apparently, it was supposed to be easy. It was part of *my* body, after all. But I remember lying in bed, touching my genitals with a degree of concern and wondering if that was it; my clitoris. I'm not sure what I expected it to feel like, or what the qualifications for my clitoris were that I was not finding. Using the words of guidance I'd heard, which formed a sort of auditory map of the external part of my genitalia, I knew my clit was definitely located somewhere near this "hood" that I'd heard described and I knew that it was higher up than the other parts of my genitals like my urethra (my pee hole, as I knew it), but still in a somewhat central location, and definitely not as far down as any openings. I felt perplexed: what if I didn't have one? Or, what if it was so small that I'd never find it? What if I was missing out on this special thing that everyone else had but me? I was anxious to know where this thing was, now that I knew I was supposed to have one. I became worried.

Sometime later, after more conversations with my mom and other adults about the specifics of this body part, I was lying in bed at night touching this bump and thinking to myself, this must be it. It seemed tiny and almost insignificant after all that concern. Putting my finger up against that tiny spot under that flap of skin deemed the "hood," I did what would later become a signature gesture of mine: I picked at it. Pain shot through me and the relief at finding it was replaced with a sudden fear that I'd accidentally picked off my own clitoris. Unsure, I consulted my mom the next day to be sure, and through my descriptions, I got confirmation that not only had I found my clit, but there was no way I'd accidentally removed it with my own fingernail. I was instantly relieved and walked away with a newfound sense of confidence and accomplishment.

When I was a teenager, I certainly did not want to talk about masturbation or my clitoris. Nothing could kill a conversation like the mention of masturbation. But when I was a little kid, I was blatantly curious. As I referenced earlier, I had entire conversations with my mom about where my clitoris was located because I wanted to know for sure that I had the right part identified. I would masturbate on my teddy bears and in the hot tub, or anywhere I felt like. My sister and I would even collaborate over which water jet made us feel the best. I didn't have a label for it, I just did what felt right.

But when I started puberty, masturbation was off-limits. It's not like I didn't do it; in fact, I masturbated a lot more often as a teen. It's just that I didn't want anyone to know or to ever, *ever*, talk about it in front of me. Now, my parents are human sexuality educators and I live with a group of people that have dedicated their lives to pleasurable living. It's not like I was on the hot seat every day about masturbation, but the topic certainly came up. And each time I would full-body flush and fold up with complete and utter embarrassment. My dad actually came up with a code-word for the term: for the span of about ten years he would exclusively refer to masturbation as "the m-thing" when around my sister or me.

You may be wondering why I was raised in an environment where not only did we talk about masturbation, but we actually had a code word for it so that my parents would be able to bring it up with me in a way that I found more palatable. It's a good question: masturbation is hardly a socially acceptable activity. Historically, there have been philosophers, religious leaders, political influencers, and all kinds of people who commented on masturbation, but the tide didn't truly turn to the negative until the early 1700s when a religious movement began proclaiming masturbation as a form of "self-pollution."[1] Many myths around masturbation have existed and been spread rampantly: that you'll go blind, your palms will grow hair, and on and on.

Personally, I am reluctant to delve too deeply into the negative history around masturbation, mainly because there's absolutely nothing wrong with it, so what's the point in discussing the negative attitudes people have had around the subject? Michael Patton, a scholar who studies masturbation (oh yes, that exists!), said that "there has been no other form of sexual activity that has been more frequently discussed, more roundly condemned, and more universally practiced than masturbation."[2] I include this quotation because it speaks to one of the fascinating aspects of masturbation: as much as people frown upon it, those same people are most likely going home and having a good, long masturbation session after they get done with all that frowning because, survey says, just about everybody does it.[3] But I appreciate the fact that we are not masturbating in a bubble: we are influenced by the thoughts and views of the people, media, and laws surrounding us. So I'm here to tell you, once and for all, that masturbation is good, pleasurable, and completely harmless.

Masturbation is a natural part of life and is part of being a human, and the overwhelming majority of people have done it at *least* once.[4] Plus, you can't discount the lie factor or people's varying definitions of what masturbation is. In case you're wondering precisely what I mean by this term, to masturbate is to touch your own genitals for pleasure. It's just you, your hands, your body parts, and the mission to create pleasure in your body.

My parents taught my sister and I to feel good about our bodies and to make sure we enjoyed them. Earlier when I referenced how my parents would bring up the "m-thing" with my sister and I, they wanted to make masturbation something we *could* talk about, since to them it didn't need to be off-limits or a taboo topic. So, they ensured that we got to see sex as a normal and important part of life as a human. Over time, this conversation grew and shifted as we aged, matured, and became interested in different aspects of our bodies. When I was a kid, I was curious about my body and felt good about exploring and figuring out about how all my parts worked, so I asked a lot of questions. Early on, my mom told me what masturbation was and how it was a way to feel pleasure in my body. When I was a teenager, I began to learn about masturbation as a tool.

Masturbation is part of being a sensing human being. We have five basic senses of which touching is an integral part of our life experience. We gather information through touch by assessing the texture, moisture, and temperature of the people and items we come into contact with. We use touch to get things done: moving objects to different positions, bringing possessions to others, handing items to one another. We use touch on ourselves to primp, to scratch, to assess, and to pleasure. There are many ways that we take pleasure from touch in our daily lives, from showering in the morning to the sensation of a book page under our fingertips. We greet friends, family, and sometimes acquaintances with a moment of equal full-body contact, a funny act that we call "hugging." We choose clothes, bedding, and even building materials for how they feel against our skin. Taking pleasure, even the smallest, seemingly indistinguishable amount, is an everyday addition to our experience as we move through the world.

There are many simple ways to begin experiencing pleasure from our bodies within these everyday experiences. Washing my hair, for example, is a daily opportunity that I can take advantage of. Setting just the right water temperature so that it's right on the edge of too hot but still easy against my skin, combined with that initial sensation of water meeting dry hair, is the first sensing combination of any shower. Selecting my favorite shampoo and taking in the burst of tea tree oil that escapes upon snapping open the lid comes next. Pouring a small pool of cool shampoo in my palm, I rub my hands together while anticipating the scrubbin' to come. Immersing my hair in suds and palms, I set to work scratching and rubbing with my fingertips from the front of my hairline to the back, ensuring that my whole head feels worked over and refreshed. Rinsing next, the heat makes my scalp tingle and a quick pat with my hands determines that my hair has changed texture. The follicles are newly individual and feel squeaky and shiny under the pad of each finger. In this rather mundane activity of getting my hair clean, there have been hundreds of sensing experiences. Most, if not all, were ones that I categorized as pleasurable.

If we take pleasure from hair washing, why not from other parts of the body as well? We were all born with particular areas of our bodies that are especially sensitive. Some of these areas, like our nipples, lips, or genitalia, are referred to as "erogenous zones." (For more specific information about how these specific areas function and can be experienced pleasurably, please refer to chapter 2 on anatomy.) But whether or not an area has been officially deemed "erogenous" or even especially sensitive, you can still experience pleasure there. Earlobes, the insides of our elbows, and nose tips have all been reported as areas from which we can experience great sensation.

Deliberately taking time in your day to appreciate these different areas can be a positive addition to your life. While applying your face lotion, take a pause to take in the curvature of your cheekbones, the softness of your cheeks, or the rough stubble you may find. While pulling on a pair of leggings or pants, appreciate the firmness of the fabric against the curvature of your legs. These tiny moments of appreciation add to creating a sense of enjoyment.

All of these are a form of self-pleasure, and masturbation is no different. Masturbation is simply the stimulation of one's own genitals. It's stimulating this specific part of your body that contains a plethora of nerve endings and has a great potential for pleasure. Approaching masturbation from this viewpoint completely reworks our standard narrative around this part of human behavior. There is simply no room for negativity within this framework. Clitorises, penises, scrotums, labia, nipples, and earlobes are body parts we're born with, simple as that. Enjoying each part for what it is and exploring its potential for sensation and pleasure is part of leading a full, sensing life. And if it makes you feel better, extensive research has concluded that there are many positive attributes from masturbation, including (but not limited to) releasing tension and experiencing increased positivity around sexuality as a whole.[5]

I masturbated long before I knew that masturbation was a thing. When I was four or five years old I recall straddling one of my favorite teddy bears, the brown one with the off-white face and short, tufty, hair and wrestling my body all over it. Simply put, it just felt *great* in my body to do that, even if I had no clue as to the mechanics of what was happening; I didn't think to myself "I'm masturbating," but I knew that what I was doing felt good. I would have just kept on wrestling and rubbing and rolling on and on, lost in my own world, but I was suddenly interrupted by my sister on the next bed who asked me what I was up to. Caught, I stopped mid-straddle and laid flat on the bear before replying, "nothing." In that moment, I became aware that this activity was something just for me. I knew that I'd return to that teddy bear soon enough, this time without my sister there to ask questions.

Masturbation has continued to be part of my life since that early experience. And while teddy bears aren't my current go-to, that first time certainly wasn't the last time. A year or so later, my sister and I discovered hot tub jets, which was a new level of masturbation comprehension. And still later, when I was a teenager and making my way through puberty, I started to become aware of the way the energy was changing in my body. I'd begun experiencing big swings in my emotions; in the morning when I woke I might feel happy and chipper, but a small incident had the potential to set me off. That's when I began to use masturbation as a way to enjoy my body and to get into agreement with the changes and increase in energy I was experiencing.

As a teen, there were many outlets and uses for the energy I would experience in my body. Sometimes it would take the form of a long run, or a particularly successful and gratifying soccer practice. Other times, it would look like getting really upset with my friends or my parents. I'd get worked up over small details that were anything but small at the time. Once I stormed out of the house to find my friend who'd read a postcard that I wanted to mail. I yelled at her and called her a bitch for invading my privacy. I can still see the stunned look on her face as she sat eating lunch and chewing on a chicken bone. This increase of energy would at times make me feel out of control.

As I've grown, I've found that there is an alternative to being at the mercy of my emotions, which is through deliberately taking care of myself. One of the ways I do this is through masturbation.

There are all sorts of ways to masturbate: with your hands, with a finger, with a sex toy, with water, or of course: rubbing yourself on a teddy bear (to name a few). I strongly encourage everyone to explore their body in whatever way suits them. Taking time to pay attention to your body is important, it's healthy, it feels good, and it's key to leading a pleasurable life.

You can use masturbation as a tool for getting to know your own body. Since you are the one running the show, you can take time to examine your genitalia and find out what pleasures you. By using different pressures, touching different areas, and by looking at your genitals directly, you can find out what you like. What you find pleasurable may change day by day—for instance one morning you may like lighter pressure, but by the evening you may find you like firmer pressure. You can regularly check in with your body by masturbating and discovering what feels good in that moment.

There are a couple of especially effective ways of masturbating. The one at the top of my list is digitally with your finger(s). Your finger is a precise touching instrument; with all of those thousands of nerve endings available to you, it makes sense to use the best tool that you've got.[6] I prefer to use the index finger of my right hand to stroke my clitoris directly, with the aid of my thumb on my right hand which I use to push my hood back and stabilize my clitoris. You can also use your other hand to help pull the hood back. With the palm of your left hand you can gently press the upper part of your mons back which will lift the clitoral hood, making the glans more accessible.

Everyone's genitals are different; some women's clitorises are covered completely by their hood and some are more prominent, just as some penises are more prominent or are covered with a foreskin. Genitals come in a rainbow of colors, textures, and shapes. There isn't a better or worse; this is about finding out what you've got and exploring your body to find out what you like.

And, keep in mind, what suits you can and does change. When I was eight years old and couldn't find my clitoris, I didn't realize that the geography and shape of my genitals would not stay the same. I figured that my vulva would get bigger as the rest of my body did, but that'd be about it. Everything grows, sensational parts shift, and there are always changes occurring.

I highly recommend looking at your genitals with a hand mirror. Find a mirror and a private space and look around down there. Go into the experience with a non-critical eye, like what was discussed in chapter 2. This is very important: leave all of the judgment and doubt at the door and decide to simply research. What does the clitoris or apex actually look like? What color are the inner labia or shaft? By being inquisitive instead of judgmental, you're creating a winning experience for yourself. Note changes that happen throughout your time looking in the mirror. Are colors changing? Have parts of your genitals changed shape or size? You can do this regularly and you may find changes that happen over the course of weeks, months, and years.

For masturbation, I recommend a lubricant because it aids in exploration and sensation. Without a lubricant, chafing may occur. Since you're taking the time to masturbate, you might as well set yourself up for success and the greatest amount of pleasure. (Please refer to the Resources chapter for the best kind of lubricants to use for masturbation.) Before you start, take a moment to smooth back any hairs that are around your clitoris or base of your penis.

Once you decide to begin masturbating, I recommend pulling back your hood and touching your clitoris directly so that you can fully access your whole clitoral glans. Try using up-and-down strokes with medium pressure to begin. I call this the "bread and butter stroke" because it's a good, reliable type of stroke that I highly recommend to anyone. Go from there and find out what you like. You can experiment with pressure, speed, length of stroke, and anything else you can think of!

For those of my readers who have a penis, you can also use the bread and butter stroke. You can curve and wrap your hand around the head to maximize the amount of contact with your apex, glans, and urethral canal, as those are the most sensitive areas of the penis. By ensuring you are stroking those areas, you will create a more pleasurable experience for yourself. If you have a foreskin, you can pull back the skin and hold it with your other hand to expose the most sensitive part of your penis. You can use a medium-length, medium-pressured stroke that emphasizes those sensitive areas. Once you have developed a steady stroke, you can research from there what you like by varying the length, speed, and pressure.

Masturbation doesn't have to be goal-oriented. When our society talks about sex, we often use terms of production. The goal is to orgasm, to ejaculate, to go over the edge, to cum/come—whatever you like to call it. That aspect of masturbation can definitely be a lot of fun. Yet, there is another way. You can go into the experience with an open mind without necessarily focusing on producing a climax. You may end up feeling a lot more sensation. Remember to take your time and make feeling a priority. Doing what feels good to you is a winning model of sensuality. Being guided by your pleasure, by what you feel in your body, only results in more pleasure.

If you begin to figure out what you like, entire worlds of sensation will open up to you. For example, you may find that one side or area of your clitoris is more sensitive than other parts, and then the next day, that same spot may feel totally different. By having feeling and sensation be a priority, you open yourself up to new experiences. You can also find out more about what you like and then communicate about it with a partner when (and if) you decide that's what you want. In the words of famed sex educator Betty Dodson, "sexual skills are like any other skills; they're not magically inherited, they have to be learned."[7] To that point, it is difficult to know what to ask for in a sensual experience if you don't have a foundation already in place. Through exploring your body and deliberately building pleasure in it, you will have a clearer idea of what to ask for and what to create in experiences with another person.

Fantasy

I have more to say about taking a pleasure-oriented approach to sensual experiences in the following chapter, but for now let's talk about another fun aspect of our bodies: fantasy. Fantasy is what happens in your mind that you imagine happening, it doesn't always have to do with real life or anything that you actually want to have happen. It can be sexual but that's not always true; sometimes when lingering in bed in the morning I fantasize about the cup of tea I'm going to make for myself when I get up. Conceptual thought is one of your senses; it's your mind at play. Everyone fantasizes and there is no point in judging yourself on what or how you fantasize, despite how crazy you might think your fantasies are.

I first remember fantasizing when I was about six or seven. I had this idea that people could eat food out of each other's genitals; it must have been one of my early formulations of what sex meant. These imaginings would get pretty elaborate: entire sandwiches complete with condiments and sliced meat would be stored inside of a person only to come out, ready to be consumed by the other person. In retrospect, perhaps I stumbled upon the term "eating pussy," and that was all I could do to make sense of it. There's no use in trying to figure out *why* I thought about that, I just did. I'd lay in bed, gazing off into the distance imagining this act taking place, adding more foods in when I deemed appropriate, all the while the core of my body continued heating up and the good feelings spread through me.

When I was eight I had these very raunchy fantasies about two blonde women making out. The details are fuzzy but if you pictured two fit and fake-tanned professional wrestler-types going at it on top of one another, that's what the fantasy looked like. I don't know how much actual sex was going on but picturing these women rolling around together was captivating. It also worried me. I figured since I had these good feelings from picturing women that it made me a lesbian. I approached my mom one afternoon while she was weeding our front garden bed and, after some hemming and hawing, asked if I was correct in my conclusion. She gave me a puzzled look and said "no." So I walked away, slightly relieved, and ready to get back to my blonde-wrestler sexcapades.

There are so many negative messages in our culture about sex, that even thinking about it seems wrong. But I say go for it, think about whatever it is that turns you on; it doesn't mean that you want to do it. Fantasy can be a fun way to turn your body on and it doesn't have to mean anything more than that.

There are two main types of fantasy. The first type is akin to a Rolodex; a series of images that you like or turn you on. Maybe it's a particular body part on a man or woman, or a feeling or sensation you had during a sensual experience. Tossing and turning in bed as a teenager, I would replay over and over again the moment right before I kissed a particular boy that I liked; it was an intense, hovering moment mixed with tension and a building of sensation that inevitably climaxed when my lips touched his soft, inviting mouth. I'd replay that frame over and over again before finally succumbing to sleep.

Another type of fantasy tells more of a story. Sometimes when I'm fantasizing, I will spend most of my time creating the setting for the sensual act to take place: the location, who is there, what they're wearing, what I'm wearing, what the room we are in looks like, etcetera. Sometimes those details are what turn me on the most, and the part about making out plays a secondary role. And on other days, I'll develop extensive plots containing a variety of different sex acts with a variety of different people that interweave and build upon one another. There's a huge range when it comes to fantasizing.

Fantasy and masturbation are both natural parts of being human; regardless of your sexual preference, gender identity, or cultural upbringing. Both utilize aspects of the senses we are born with: conceptual thought and touch. By deliberately adding pleasure to your life through masturbation, you have a tool for creating a better experience. You can use masturbation as a way to change your mindset or simply take a break. When you are experiencing a lot of energy in your body, you can masturbate as a way to experience that increase of energy pleasurably. Similarly, when you are experiencing low energy, you can get into agreement with that, too, by choosing to create pleasure in your body. Too often we are told that sex is wrong or something to be embarrassed about. You can change the conversation by intentionally appreciating your own body and giving yourself pleasure.

Chapter 6
THE BIG "O"

Too often, orgasm (or more broadly, pleasurable, fun sex) is relegated to a final chapter in sex education books, or not discussed at all. To make matters worse, when talking directly to teens, the subject is skipped even more often due to the ageist, Puritanical social rules of our society. The only conversation we should be having with teenagers is about how to have a good sex life, because let's be honest, most already know plenty about the mechanics through porn or social media outlets. Your average sex ed class in high school (if it's offered at all) probably isn't going to tell you anything you didn't already know about how sex works.

As a whole, we mainly talk about sex in a way that is problem-oriented and lacking in solutions. With young women, we tell them that their first time having intercourse will be painful and that they could be exposed to STIs (sexually transmitted infections). With adults, we usually hear people talk about what's wrong; their partner takes too long to orgasm, their partner doesn't orgasm at all, or there is a complete lack of sex. It's all about what isn't working or what isn't happening.

Speculating about why all this negativity about sex exists is a whole 'nother book entirely and is simply beyond the scope of my project. Part of it is cultural; I'm making pretty broad statements about how people talk about sex here in America, but people from other parts of the world treat sex differently. Some countries, like France and the Netherlands, have much more comprehensive sex education and have generally more liberal views on sexuality, which results in fewer unplanned pregnancies and lower rates of STIs.[1]

Generally speaking, America simply doesn't do sex education very well. Despite the fact that public health researchers have concluded pleasure-inclusive sex education is effective in reducing the potential negative consequences of sexual activity (like STIs), there has been difficulty integrating that viewpoint into the public curriculum.[2] Hence, the United States has higher rates of teen pregnancy and STIs in comparison to other developed countries.[3] Overall, youth are not getting the information needed in order to have pleasurable, healthy sex lives as adults. This is not just a US issue: a recent UK study demonstrated that half the young women surveyed couldn't properly identify their reproductive anatomy[4] and a later study by the same group showed that men fared similarly when identifying female anatomy.[5] If people are unable to name basic and essential parts of each other's bodies, how can we be expected to know how to pleasure others, let alone pleasure ourselves?

We exist in a culture that values pain over pleasure. Popular slogans like "no pain, no gain" are examples of this emphasis. When we read the news or watch it on TV, we are mainly told who suffered the most amount of pain that day, summed up by the notion "if it bleeds, it leads." One example of this is how we consume news: of the top fifteen stories of 2012, over half were about pain (deaths) and an additional fifth had to do with financial crisis.[6] It's not to say that these are not important aspects of our lives, but there is certainly an imbalance.

Not only do we value pain, but we're actually perceiving ourselves as experiencing larger amounts of it than the rest of the world. According to a recent study, people in the United States, Australia, and Great Britain report experiencing more pain than the other twenty-seven countries surveyed, up to four times that of the countries reporting experiencing the least pain.[7] Furthermore, the United States, Canada, and Western Europe consume the vast majority of opioids, approximately 95 percent of all opioids available on the global market[8] (with America alone consuming a whopping 80 percent of all opioids).[9] There is a huge emphasis on pain in our culture: from the medical industry to our personal life philosophies.

The conversation about sexuality has already begun to shift. With the sexual revolution in the sixties and seventies, we have seen a lot of change. And more currently, there has been much more discussion in mainstream media about sex and creating more equality between the sexes. As a result, we're beginning to open up the collective conversation around human sexuality and pleasure. As an example: orgasm is a hot topic in the current culture. You can read secrets to successfully experiencing an orgasm from magazines displayed next to chewing gum at the register of your local grocery store. There are more blogs, websites, and small businesses dedicated to helping people with their sex lives (read: achieve orgasm regularly) than you can shake a stick at. Non-fiction books offer advice, novels hint at its existence, and movies demonstrate the mystical fireworks nature of the experience. Not to mention pornography, which is widely available and offers (unrealistic) portrayals of how orgasm and sex itself works.

Before we delve further into a pleasure-oriented approach to orgasm, it's time to talk about the clitoris. If you happened to skip chapter 2 on anatomy, please refer to that chapter for a fuller exploration of this particularly important part of a vulva. The clitoris was actually edited out of *Grey's Anatomy* (the standard source of all things anatomy in the twentieth century) between 1901–1946 and it took Helen O'Connell's groundbreaking MRIs of the entire clitoris in 2005 to finally show the world what the clitoris is all about.[10]

The reason I keep emphasizing the clitoris is because it's the source of all female orgasm. The sole function of the clitoris is pleasure: we do not urinate, have babies, or defecate from our clitoris. Many other parts of our bodies have nerve endings which can be taken advantage of for our pleasure, but the clitoris is the only one that's just there for our own enjoyment. The clitoris can be very sensitive: there are over eight thousand pressure sensitive nerve endings in the glans, which is a relatively small surface area in the external portion of the vulva. The penis has just as many nerve endings, but they're spread out over the glans and shaft of the penis. To that point, the glans of the clitoris has a concentration of nerve endings fifty times that of the penis, due to it's relatively smaller size.[11] O'Connell's MRI scans of the early nineties demonstrated that the clitoris is not just the glans we can see externally, but is actually made up of different parts: mainly, the clitoral bulbs and the crura which form the clitoral glans.[12]

There have been many myths historically about where female orgasm comes from and if it exists at all, but I'm here to tell you that not only does it exist, but it's based in the clitoris. Since we can now understand visually (not just through our own personal experience) that the clitoris has a larger, internal network, it's important to learn about how it functions so that those of us with vulvas can take advantage of all those nerve endings as much as we want to.

There are many ways to touch a clitoris and I trust that through doing your own research, you can find the way that feels best to you. There are often reports of people's clitorises being too sensitive or not sensitive enough, but I am of the belief that every clit can be touched just right. In the previous chapter we discussed techniques for masturbation and at the end of this chapter I'll describe a method of stroking both penises and vulvas for the greatest amount of pleasure.

· · · · · ·

But first, let's talk about orgasm.

The standard definition of orgasm describes a discharge or release of sensation at the end of a sexual cycle, usually characterized by rhythmic muscular contractions in a person's genitals. William Masters and Virginia Johnson, pioneers of sexuality as a field of research, developed a model of orgasm in the 1960s which they called "sexual response." Sexual response is a series of phases that happen when someone becomes aroused or engages in sexually stimulating activities, like masturbation or intercourse. Masters and Johnson broke this cycle down into four main parts: excitement, plateau, orgasm, and resolution. Each stage describes a part of the building or waning of sensation, of which orgasm is the peak, or moment of greatest sensation. While the cycle of sexual response can vary, the orgasm portion is a few seconds long and usually consists of fewer than ten contractions in the genital area.[13]

Here you can take a look at this cycle, or model of orgasm, graphed out:

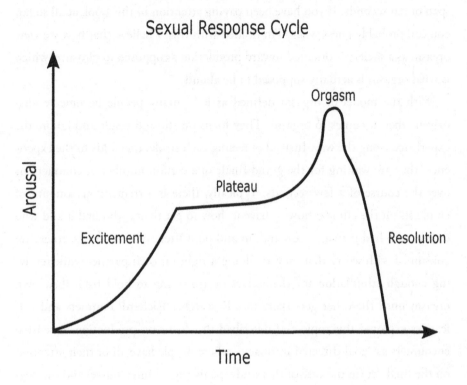

In this model of orgasm, the entire cycle is focused around that one big peak at the end. The sensation leading up to it is directed toward the goal of "orgasm," those signature series of contractions. And that is also supposed to be the most sensational point of the entire experience. As you can see in the graph, the sensation decreases dramatically after the orgasm and usually there is less sensation at the end (in the resolution phase) than in the beginning.

This model of orgasm is functional but is also very limiting. Dr. Elizabeth Gunther and Paula Spencer, authors of the enormously helpful and illuminating book on all-things vulva and vaginal, *The V Book*, use the Masters and Johnson model of orgasm in their book to begin their discussion of orgasm; however, they stipulate that "this model also levels the differences among individual women. In fact, all women are not the same, and their sexual needs, satisfactions, and problems don't fit into neat categories."[14] From what I can tell, we have a much broader range of experience than a few firm contractions over the span of ten seconds. If you have been paying attention in this book at all so far, you can probably guess where I'm headed with this: I believe that how we view orgasm as a society is oriented toward production as opposed to pleasure, which is what orgasm is actually supposed to be about!

With the model of orgasm defined as it is, many people become results-driven when it comes to orgasm. They focus on the end result and ignore the experience along the way. Instead of feeling each stroke that adds to the experience, they are waiting for the grand finale of a certain number of contractions over the course of a few seconds. Typically, there is a tremendous amount of emphasis on the climax: how to have it, how to get there, who had it and who didn't, who had it first . . . on and on and on. Often, one or both partners are consumed with worry that they are doing it right for their partner while receiving enough stimulation for themselves or are trying to hold back their own orgasm until the other gets there too. Researcher Richard Timmers and colleagues explored this topic and described this focus on production in sensual encounters as "goal-directed intimacy," where people have all of their attention on the final act (in the case of this study, penis-vagina intercourse) and the negative effects this viewpoint has on people's sex lives.[15] Orgasm and sex become a very complicated battle and, ultimately, neither partner is fully able to put their attention on what they are feeling.

What's fascinating to me is that this tendency we have as a culture toward production is apparent in the very language we use. According to the *Oxford English Dictionary*, the word orgasm originally meant "a surge of sexual excitement" or "the rut."[16] Both of these aspects of the definition relate to an experience or an *aspect* of an experience. A surge of sexual excitement could occur once, twice, or many times in an experience. The rut refers to *estrus*, a period of time in which certain mammals are fertile, or able to get pregnant. To the point, this definition of orgasm refers to a state of being or an ongoing length of time. However, the word later changes to mean "the highest point of sexual excitement."[17] This new definition marks orgasm as something that happens at one point, it's now something that can be graphed on an x-y coordinate of sensation whereas previously it was a peak of sensation or an ongoing state. While that is convenient from a research standpoint, it's not the only way people are capable of experiencing orgasm.

Orgasm does not need to be goal-oriented in the way that it has become in our society. From what I can tell, Masters and Johnson needed to break down orgasm in a way that would fit into a clinical model; something that they could monitor and collect data about. While their contribution to science and our understanding of human sexuality is enormous and I think we all are rather indebted to them for their ability and determination to research the topic of orgasm at a time when that was not socially acceptable, it is time to grow beyond this model. We're not in a lab, and no one is wearing electronic sensors for energy and body heat. Orgasm and, more broadly, human sensuality is much more complicated, intense, and interesting than something that can be broken down into four stages and monitored on a graph.

Culturally, the definition of orgasm has begun to broaden. Leading researcher Dr. Sharon Moalem, author of *How Sex Works*, describes orgasm in a way that is far more conceptual than we'd normally encounter in the mainstream perception of orgasm. He stipulates that many women can orgasm without direct genital stimulation; they experience orgasm through stimulation of other erogenous zones (like nipples or lips, for example) or through stimulating their minds, known as *conceptual thought*. Since orgasm can occur in different parts of the body, not just the genitals, Moalem stipulates that orgasm is something that we *perceive*, and that perception varies widely from person to person.[18] It's not just an automated response, it's a "state of mind."[19] If we start to think of orgasm as a conceptual experience, then we can begin to loosen up the way we perceive it as a whole.

One of the troubles with how we typically perceive orgasm is that climax (that's the ten or so contractions over a few seconds) and orgasm are thought of as being synonymous, but they're not. Climax can be a lot of fun, I like it as much as the next person. But the part leading up to a high peak, the sensation on the other side of a peak, and the sensation when coming down can all be just as intense and complex as that sought-after climax.

I think that orgasm is when your genitals feel better than any other place on your body. If you are willing to view orgasm that way, you'll have a lot more fun. We'll talk more about this later.

So now that we've explored a notion of orgasm that is focused on pleasure instead of producing a climax, I'd like to take a look at a particular kind of sex that is entirely focused on pleasure: DOing (Deliberate Orgasm). Using the definition of orgasm that I described earlier (remember: it's when your genitals feel better than any other part of your body), this is a kind of sex that prioritizes orgasm and the pleasure we are each capable of experiencing.

Chapter 7

HOW DO YOU DO?: CREATING A DELIBERATE ORGASM

What is sex?

Now that I've spent the entire last chapter convincing you that orgasm is way more than we typically think of it, I don't think the next thing I have to say will surprise you all that much. So here it is, the big news flash of the chapter: *sex might not be exactly what we think it is.* That is, just like with orgasm and masturbation, sex is much more expansive than how it's typically represented in our culture.

Often, when people use the word "sex," they mean intercourse, especially intercourse between a man and a woman (or, penis and vagina intercourse, often referred to as P-V). This usage can be seen everywhere from soap operas to magazine stands. The good ol' *Oxford English Dictionary* even falls into this trap: their definition of "sex" specifies the word as having to do with intercourse and copulation. Not only is this a *heteronormative* way of approaching sex, but the definition of sex can actually be much broader than we tend to use it in popular language. Heather Corinna simply defines sex as "consensually engaging in sexual activities with someone else."[1] This broader definition is far more inclusive and expansive than we typically use it. She elaborates further that sex can include a kissing session, fingering and hand jobs, fantasizing aloud, showing your naked body, any kind of penetrative sex in any orifice, or really anything *you* define as sex. As she so deftly describes, "you can define sex for yourself, and only you can really come up with your own lived-experience, just-your-own-self definition of what being sexual is for you. Only we can define, for ourselves, what is or isn't an expression of our sexuality."[2] I appreciate her view on sex because it encourages us to keep our mind open as to what sex can look like. This is right in line with what we've discussed previously about not needing to be goal-oriented in terms of our sensual and sexual experiences.

In a previous chapter I talked a lot about how masturbation, or more broadly any form of self-pleasure, can be approached from a pleasure-oriented view. That is, we don't need to go into a sensual experience with a particular goal in mind. Emphasizing the goal, or being results driven,[3] is sort of like wearing blinders on the sides of your head: you might be able to see straight in front of you, but you're certainly missing a lot of the view. Similarly, we can approach sex by being open to whatever pleasure is available and experiencing enjoyment and gratification from that state.

This broad, open-ended view of sexuality is somewhat complicated by the fact that we live in what I like to politely call a "fuck-oriented culture." Remember the previous chapters where I've been going on and on about how we value pain over pleasure and production over pleasure? Well one of the ways this shows up is how much we emphasize sex (i.e., intercourse) in our advertising, movies, magazines, pharmacies, and just about everywhere you look. Sex is either directly represented or alluded to in advertisements from burgers to body wash[4] "and used to sell everything from happiness to social inclusion."[5]

Representations of sex are everywhere: online, television, social media, billboards, you name it. A recent research project of movies from 1950–2006 showed that 84 percent of movies contain sexual content.[6] Over half of eleven- to sixteen-year-olds surveyed in Britain had been exposed to explicit material online, either deliberately or through advertisement. The same survey also found that most (53 percent of boys and 39 percent of girls) viewed the depictions of sex as realistic and a portion of boys indicated that it informed their own sexual choices, and over a third of twelve- to fourteen-year-olds specified that they "wanted to copy the behavior that they'd seen."[7] Views are mixed on the negative impact of people viewing and being exposed to pornography, but it does certainly show that we're exposed to a lot of sex: we can find it anywhere.[8]

But what's shown isn't realistic and it's rarely focused on pleasure. In the movies, the couple usually fling open the bedroom door, begin grabbing at one another and stripping clothing off, and immediately begin moaning and effusing pleasure. Not only is this unrealistic but it promotes risky sexual behavior.[9] A movie character rarely, if ever, makes steps to ensure the other person gets what they want or that the sexual encounter is safe. This isn't just relegated to our movies and media; it's in how we talk to one another and in our medical experiences. Only 13 percent of OB-GYNs (obstetrician-gynecologists) ask about their patients' sexual pleasure, although over 60 percent routinely ask about their patients' sexual activities.[10] So even though most doctors in that field *do* ask about their patients' sex lives, pleasure rarely if ever comes up.

This isn't a satisfying approach to sex for everyone. Research shows that there is a literal "orgasm gap," where heterosexual men experience orgasm significantly more often than heterosexual women do: heterosexual men experience orgasm 95 percent of the time, whereas heterosexual women experience orgasm during 65 percent of sexual encounters. Interestingly, when women identify as lesbian, their experience of orgasm increases significantly to 86 percent. The same study demonstrated that people who were more likely to orgasm were also more likely to include more activities into their sensual experience, like: more positive communication (like sexy talk and loving statements), more oral sex, and new positions, to list a few. It was found that adding deep kissing, manual genital stimulation, or oral sex to P-V increased orgasm.[11] So, in summary, it's not all about intercourse if you're seeking pleasure and orgasm.

Which brings me to my next topic: pleasure and orgasm!

Deliberate Orgasm

Before you start rolling your eyes at me, I'm not trying to get you not to have sex. Don't get me wrong: intercourse can be a lot of fun. My goal here is simply to shift the direction away from the collective fear and stigma around sex and create a larger conversation about something we all know is true deep down: sex is fun. Our bodies are designed to ensure that sex is fun (why else would we have a clitoris of which the sole purpose is pleasure, after all?). It's just that if sex tends to mean intercourse, it's not necessarily the most pleasurable (or inclusive) way of going about things. Remember all that information about the clitoris being the root of female orgasm? That's where Deliberate Orgasm (DO) comes in.

One of the first sensual experiences I ever had was a DO date. A DO date is when one person puts their total attention on the other person's body to create the optimum amount of pleasurable sensation. Since the penis and the clitoris are usually the two most sensational parts of our bodies, in a DO date both people put their total attention on the most sensational part of one person's body and strokes it with their finger when touching a clitoris and with their hand when touching a penis. Know for now that DOing is the most reliable and direct way of pleasuring a partner and is also the safest form of sex with a partner. Learning how to DO is life-changing because it gives you the tools to produce orgasm and pleasure in your own body and your partner's any time you want.

There is a lot to say about DOing, but perhaps the biggest thing I'd like you to know is that it is the best way to learn about pleasure and is the most effective way to train yourself (and a partner) to have pleasurable sex. Often, people have sex for reasons other than feeling good and having fun. If you're doing something other than that in a DO date, you're not having one.

Also, DOing is the safest form of partnered sex. Remember all that scary stuff they told you in the one sex ed class your school offered? Well, if you wear latex gloves and use water-based lubricant, you are completely safe from contracting or exchanging any kind of fluids (and thus, are much safer).

It's a great way to learn. In a DO date, you get to learn about the other person and you get to learn about what you like. DOing is communication-based; you're talking the whole time and you can look each other in the eye throughout the experience. And the lights are on. As scary as that may sound to some, it can also be a lot of fun depending on how you decide to look at the situation. In my experience, having your genitals looked at, touched, and described by an approving person is truly a turn-on unlike any other.

DOing takes the mystery out of sex. Some people claim that they enjoy mystery in their lives, but when it comes to sex, mystery is pointless. Since DOing and communication go hand-in-hand (like that pun?), there is no need for mystery. Spending time aimlessly wondering how you're doing, or if your partner is even enjoying the experience, is completely useless. Asking questions, making offers, and communicating what you feel is integral to a DO date and thus eliminates all mystery.

Not only is it a lot of fun but the entire DO date experience is a deliberate one for both people involved. Since the goal of a DO date is to produce pleasure, anything that you feel is right. With other sex acts, many people go into the experience with a laundry list of sensations to have or avoid. Unspoken expectations or wants mean that you and your partner may or may not succeed and it's fifty-fifty whether or not you both leave the experience feeling good about it and gratified by what happened. But through good communication, attention, and approval, a DO date is a win-win situation for both parties involved, every time.

Through DOing you can build a friendship with another person. The actual definition of the activity (reminder: two people putting their attention on one person's body for pleasure) requires putting your attention on another person's body. Through attention, you can find out about a person. You get to know what they like, what they think, how they feel. If you're willing to do what it takes to have winning experiences with another person, you'll build a friendship with them. And who doesn't want to have sex with someone they are also friends with?

How to Get Started DOing

First, communication is as much a part of DOing as the actual sex part is. In order to create a pleasurable experience for you (and your partner), be willing to communicate and say what you want! So, the first step is to ask for a DO date. DO dates rarely "just happen." They're not the same thing that happens when someone fingers you; they're different sex acts entirely. Trust me, the risk of communicating what you desire is well worth the reward.

Second, set up a space. You'll want a private area (like your bedroom) that you'll feel comfortable in. On a bed, you can arrange several pillows: some for behind your head and two beside you so that you can have your legs supported and your DOing partner can sit on as many pillows as necessary for their comfort. You'll also want to have your supplies ready and nearby: latex gloves, water-based lubricant, a small towel to go underneath you (washcloth-sized works perfectly), and a timer or clock.*

Third, both parties get into position and get comfortable. Check out the illustrations on the following pages to see good sitting positions for DO dates. The first is where the DOer sits beside the person receiving with crossed legs, or they can sit beside you with one leg over your abdomen and the other underneath your leg. Either position is great, the second allows for more contact and the DOer can also rest the hand with which they'll be stroking against their own leg for support. Either way, make sure that they can hold their hand in a relaxed position (adding a small pillow or a folded towel under their hand or forearm may be necessary to provide support).

A note about positions: although this is a common position that can be comfortable for many people, all bodies are unique and have different requirements for comfort. This position can be altered in many ways: the addition (or subtraction) of more pillows under the sitter can help with any size differences between the two people, the addition of a small pillow under the DOer's arm can ease tension in the arm, pillows can be placed in varying ways to support the legs of both people, and the whole position can be shifted in order to include people who might not be comfortable sitting up on a bed. For example, a chair can be placed beside the bed with the person receiving the DO date positioned parallel to them, close by on the edge of the bed. Openly discussing any preferences together and reaching an agreement about what is best for you before you begin will ensure that it's a fun, comfortable experience for all parties involved.

---

* I highly recommend setting a time for DO dates, seven or ten minutes are good starting places. Setting a time creates a winning situation for both people involved: everyone knows exactly when it will be over and has agreed on how long they want the experience to go for. After the DO date is over, you can always have another!

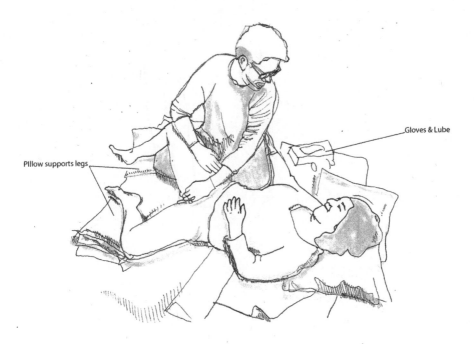

Pillow supports legs

Gloves & Lube

Next, the DOer will put on the latex gloves and add a dollop of lubricant to the index finger (for clitorises) or hand (for penises) they'll be using. Once the gloves are on, be sure that you don't touch anything else that may contaminate the gloves. With the lubricant on your hand, you can do a "lube stroke," a long stroke going from the perineum area up to their clit, or with a penis, from the base of the penis up along the shaft to the glans. Take a few moments smoothing back any hairs around their clit and labia, or away from the base of the penis—any hairs getting pulled while having a DO date *will* be felt and can cause unpleasant micro-abrasions or pulling, so this is a good thing to take care of right away.

Now you're ready to start stroking! Begin with medium pressure on the upper-left quadrant of their clitoris. Based on my experience and the information that my community teaches and researches, that is typically a sensational part of the clitoris and is a good starting place. However, always remember the age-old adage: different strokes for different folks! Please take a look at the drawing on the next page to get an idea of a good hand position for DOing (in this example: a person with a vulva). Every clitoris can be touched just right.

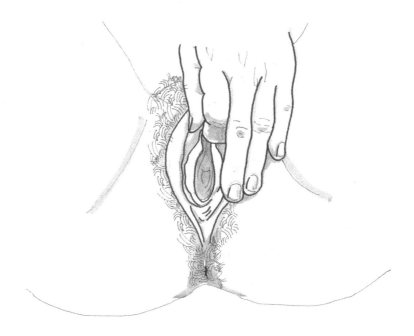

For stroking a penis, begin with medium pressure and length of stroke. Using one hand to hold the base or shaft of the penis while stroking with the other hand can be a good way to start the DO date. If uncircumcised, the hand holding the base of the penis can also be used to pull back the foreskin.

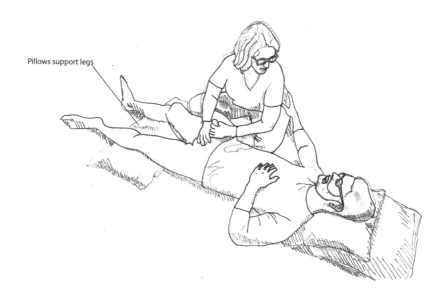

Pillows support legs

As mentioned previously, this position can be adapted for different body shapes and abilities. Ensure that both people are in a comfortable position and are well supported by pillows. For stroking a penis, make sure your hands are able to access the genital region in a relaxed, well-supported way.

From there, keep talking. Ask questions that they can answer with a "yes" or "no." For example, "would you like more pressure?" Or, "would you like a shorter stroke?" If they say yes, keep asking until you get a "no," that's when you know you've given them precisely what you're offering. You can continually make offers throughout the DO date; something they said "no" to earlier may be a "yes" later.

For the person getting DOne, they can let the person DOing them know how they're succeeding. If you like the pressure they're using, tell them! If you're really thrilled to be having this DO date with them, tell them! Letting your partner know they're succeeding makes the experience even more fun. If you'd like a change, ask in a way that is winning: something that is possible for them to do (i.e., increase the pressure) and ask for one thing at a time which will ensure that:

1. they'll hear you and understand what you want.
2. the likelihood of you getting exactly what you want will increase.

Description is a fun part of DOing. Telling your partner what their genitals look like, especially how beautiful they are, can be very pleasurable. Describing colors, shapes, and textures adds to the experience. By acknowledging what you see in an approving way, you're adding to the good feelings of the experience. A lot of people, especially those with vulvas, never look at their genitals, so having it described can be a new, potentially pleasurable, experience.

Having another person look at me and tell me what he observed was one of the most standout aspects of my first DO date. As well as the fact that it felt damn good.

Growing up in a community with a focus on sensuality didn't mean I was excused from all of the regular eccentricities we've all got about sex and our basic sexuality as humans. I just got a way, way smaller dose than most people.

All of our limitations are learned; limitations are values and boundaries we've chosen for ourselves because, when it comes right down to it, we are the ones giving them validity. This is all to say that I had my own hang ups about my body, about my pussy, and about having sex. I didn't turn eighteen and suddenly feel like some sort of sex goddess. No, I was self-conscious. I had questions. I was awkward. But what's different is that I actively decided to expand my sensuality through learning about it myself. DOing is one of the ways I learned about my body and my own capacity to experience pleasure.

I had my first DO date when I was seventeen. Before then I'd had a few assorted experiences, like kissing and late-night rolling around, but nothing beyond some rather fun, exploratory hand-genital forays. Then, one day, I decided to have my first DO date. The idea of "having a DO date" was this rather mystical experience for me. I'd heard the words "DO date" and "DOing" tossed around for years; not in a sexual way, but as a concept, like how you'd be familiar with the words "garbage truck" even if you'd never gotten up early enough to actually see the truck pull up and take away your trash with your own eyes, yet you still know it exists and what it does. So here I was, on the verge of seeing that truck up close and personal.

Max and I had never had any kind of sex together, let alone a DO date. But we both understood the mechanics of the activity and had been friends for a number of years, so I thought he was the perfect candidate for my first DO date; we were starting from a place of good feelings and no expectations. Even so, it was quite something to walk up to him one day and squeak out those initiating words, "do you want to have a DO date?"

The day of the date, I felt hot. It is that particular brand of heat that lives in your torso and has nothing to do with temperature. I had no doubt that this was the right thing to do and that it was what I wanted; it was the getting started that I felt hung up about. Even though we were in the bedroom together, fully aware of what we were about to do, I still had to ask myself: was I really about to crawl up onto my bed (I was in the top bunk) and take my pants off in front of this guy? But I did it. I ambled up there first and pulled off my pants, leaving my tank top in place. He came up after me and got into position at my side.

Again, I reminded myself that this was *really* happening. The he looked down at me with a quiet, approving smile and I realized that I could just relax.

Unclamping my legs, I spread them open to reveal my vulva. My legs felt like they made an audible creak as they parted: the last boundary to this experience actually happening. "There it is," I felt like saying. He put his gloved fingertip down and then contact was made. The coolness of the lube sunk into me and the pressure of his finger, I realized, actually felt good. This was fun.

Then he started talking. He began describing my vulva, which surprised me. Not only was he going to touch me and look at my genitalia directly, but he was going to talk about it? He described the length and coloring of my inner and outer labia and I felt this wash of approval go over me. That attention sank into my chest and has never left. The words are long gone, but the effect of having another person's approving attention directly on my body is something that has stayed with me since, many years later.

He took me on several peaks of sensation and then brought me down toward the end by using firmer, slower pressure. I realized that I felt better afterwards than when we had started. My energy had a longer, more drawn out quality to it. Before the date the inside of my body felt like a pinball machine—all bright lights and shooting sensations flooding my nervous system. But laying there on the bed afterward, I felt quiet. My body felt warm and heavy and I had a rested, gratified feeling that I found I quite liked.

It's the communication aspect of DOing that is one of the reasons I like it so much. Since I'm able (and encouraged) to talk and ask questions, there's no need for mystery between me and the person I'm having the experience with. Communication is the foundation of DOing. Both people can see each other and talk throughout the entire experience. The person getting DOne or having their genitals stroked can tell their partner what they like and what else they want. The person doing the stroking can describe any changes they may perceive (like color and texture, for example) and can ask any questions they have (like "would you like more pressure?"). Very rarely are we encouraged to talk before, during, or after sex. In fact, sex is supposed to be a pretty silent verbal affair apart from moaning. With DOing, everyone has an opportunity to learn, to get to know their partner better, and to get to know what they like so they can enjoy themselves.

And since DOing is not production-oriented, you're not trying to create just *one* experience with a set outcome. Instead, you have an opportunity to learn about the other person and to do what you know will pleasure them. You're creating the most good you possibly can for that person. Most of the time when people have sex, their goal is to orgasm or "go over," but with this kind of sex, there is no goal besides fun.

In the previous chapter, I defined orgasm as when your crotch feels better than any other part of your body. This way of viewing orgasm has led to what my community refers to as a "dome-shaped orgasm" which is in contrast to the Masters and Johnson model which, if graphed out, would be more in the shape of a staircase with an abrupt end. In the dome-shaped model, you build sensation and then back off with a "peak" or any change in the stroke. After creating a peak, you can return to the building stroke and continue creating more peaks. By creating a range of sensations, you can create a dome-shaped orgasm where you build sensation throughout the entire experience.

This graph demonstrates both models of orgasm, with the standard definition (the familiar climax-focused model within the larger graph) and the updated definition (the larger dome):

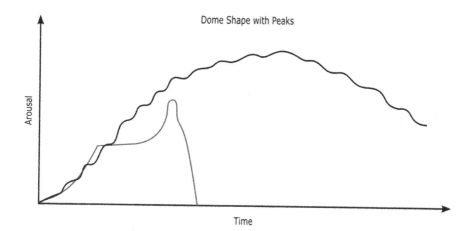

As you can see, the dome-shaped orgasm contains many peaks which builds and elongates the amount of sensation that can be felt in the entire experience. There is just as much to be felt on the other side of the peak. No "going over" or ejaculation is required, but it can be part of the experience. This is in contrast to Masters and Johnson's definition in which going over is the emphasis. The sensation completely ends as soon as ejaculation has occurred: male ejaculation marks the end of the sex act in this model of orgasm. Instead of going into a sensual experience with a set goal, like going over or having your partner go over, we can expand our minds. DOing includes a new definition of orgasm that is pleasure-based. Through altering the way we look at sexuality and sensuality, we open ourselves up to the possibility of feeling more.

This is just the tip of the iceberg (*or just the "glans" of the clitoris!* Let's make that the new analogy of choice). There is so much more to say about Deliberate Orgasm and about creating a new view of orgasm itself. And the great thing about both of these subjects is that they're expansive and are something you can keep learning more about and increasing your own understanding of throughout your life. DOing is a great way to start off having sex because you get so much information right alongside your pleasure. It's unique in its pleasure-forward structure. This form of sexing is more like that hot cup of Earl Grey tea in the handmade mug; it's taking in your senses and feeling what there is to feel in the moment.

I also appreciate the inclusive format of this form of sex. As I mentioned earlier, the positions of DO dates can be altered depending on who wants to do what and what each body is capable of. DOing is great for same-sex partners, heterosexual people, gender non-conforming, and for people not interested in sex but who are interested in masturbating, as the principals of DOing can be applied to masturbation. With DOing, the focus is on paying attention and using your intention to create the most amount of sensation possible—that's the important part. We are a spectrum of bodies, preferences, and particularities and through open communication, we can learn to give each other what we want as well as have the experiences we want to have. DOing and DO dates are just more tools in your (sensuality) belt.

Now that you're all revved up and ready to give it a whirl, here are ten steps to having a DO date:

Ten Steps of a DO Date

1. Ask your friend if they'd like to have a DO date and arrange the when/where.

This can be very simple, whether or not you've had a DO date with them before. If you have, the groundwork has already been set. If you haven't, you could explain briefly how a DO date is set up and that it's a no-strings-attached opportunity for fun and research. You could even show them this list: keep it simple!

2. Set up your space.

Make sure that you have a private, safe area so that you can both relax. Have your supplies (latex gloves, lubricant, towel, and clock or timer) nearby.

3. Arrange yourselves on the bed.

The person DOing usually sits to the side (either right or left) of the person being stroked. If it's a person with a vulva receiving the DO date, they will have their legs opened and relaxed, and they can support their thighs with a pillow. If it's a person with a penis getting DOne, they will lay flat with their legs slightly open, and they can support their legs with pillows as well. The person DOing can sit on a pillow. Put a small towel under the person being DOne, so it'll be there for wiping off at the end and to catch any fluids.

4. Put on your gloves and apply the lubricant.

Tell your partner what you're going to do before you do it. Put a generous dollop of lube (nickel-sized) on your finger tip if you'll be touching a clit, or a small puddle (silver dollar-sized) if you'll be touching a penis. With firm but gentle pressure, apply the lubricant. This is the first time you'll be touching them directly, so go slow and be deliberate.

5. Set up your hand position.

If you're touching a clitoris, anchor the thumb of the hand you'll be stroking with next to their clit in order to stabilize it, and put your other hand under their butt to create another point of contact.

If you're touching a penis, you can use one hand to hold the base of their penis while you use your other hand to stroke. Later, you can always decide to use one hand, but this can be a nice way to start off.

6. Start stroking!

In the beginning you may want to use firmer, slower strokes. When you feel like the sensation is rolling, or if your partner communicates that they would like a change, you can lighten up and use your intention to build sensation.

7. Peak your partner.

Using a consistent stroke will build steady sensation in the person you're touching. You can peak them by making a change—like slowing down, increasing pressure, or pausing. Any change in pressure, speed, or length of stroke will create a peak.

8. Bring them down.

At the end of your DO date, you can bring your partner down with slower strokes and increased pressure. Much like at the beginning of the DO date, this is grounding. This is a good time to be talking! You can tell your partner how you liked the change in pressure, or that you'd like more pressure. And if you're the one DOing, you can report any changes you notice, like: color, engorgement, sensations, or anything else! The sky's the limit.

9. Towel them off.

Since you used plenty of lubricant, and more fluids may or may not have been produced during the experience, you can use the towel that was underneath them to wipe off any excess moisture. It's a nice thing to do and can feel very good. Use firm, solid pressure and do not (*do not*) dab at them.

10. Tell them how fun it was.

With DOing, you can communicate throughout the entire experience. At the end, it's fun to acknowledge a specific moment that felt particularly good or stood out to you.

Chapter 8

SAFE SEX AND ALL ABOUT LATEX

Safer Sex

When I was eleven and starting to get into the swing of puberty, I was very curious about oral sex. Specifically, oral sex on a penis. This was long before I had any sexual or sensual experiences with someone other than myself, but I was obsessed with the sex act as a concept. I knew that people enjoyed it (why else would this activity exist? I'd ask myself), but it seemed totally improbable to me. All of it: the how, the why, the when. The mouth touching the penis. It simply didn't compute and the notion that it could possibly be fun for other people was downright puzzling: it seemed like a recipe for discomfort for both parties. It wasn't like I thought about oral sex every day, but when I did, I was pretty worked up about it. Suffice it to say, I felt intensely curious and wanted to know how to pleasurably approach the experience when the time came.

Fast forward a couple of years. I still didn't have any answers. I continued pondering the total absurdity of the act and hypothesizing that I'd be terrible at it and never wanting to try it. Whenever I got up the courage to query my adult friends about it, they'd usually smile at me and find some way to avoid my questions.

Around that time, when my sister and I first started writing the precursor to this book, our friend who was moderating the project gave us writing prompts on subjects having to do with sex education. Number one on the list was oral sex, and she suggested that we write about whatever it was we knew or thought we knew about oral sex as a way of describing the concept and potentially explaining it to a reader. The topic was open-ended and we had the option of skipping it if we wanted to. But, I took this particular prompt quite personally and typed back, in a jumbled mixture of all-caps and dozens of exclamation points, "how could you ask me about this! You know this is something I have questions about! Ahhh!" Face flushed and mind swimming, I was upset. I sat at our desk in the main office—fluorescent bulbs overhead, the wood pellet stove's cacophony ringing in the background—and wrote out my hurried response at our shared desktop computer, personally offended and on the verge of tears at the mere mention of "oral sex." Clearly, this was a topic I had a lot of questions about.

Later that year, while a group of us were perusing a gigantic Barnes and Noble book store, I snuck off from the group to do my own research. I'd come across the Adult Education aisle before and I suspected it might contain some answers. I picked up a random book that looked likely and flipped through until I found a section on oral sex on a man. Quietly and intently, I scoped the chapter trying to glean as much as I could about the mechanics and function of this particular sex act. I nearly shot out of my skin when my Mom tapped me on my shoulder a few minutes into my reading. I shoved the book back on the shelf and tried to act cool, like I'd just wandered in there and really had no idea what was going on. She asked me what I'd been reading about and I squeezed out the words to tell her. In a few short, mumbled sentences I told her that I wanted to know about oral sex, how it worked, and about how climax fit into that whole situation. She told me, firmly, that I didn't ever have to be ashamed about that, that it was not only fine to be curious, but that it was perfectly natural. The slightly puzzled but approving look that she gave me while I peered up at her while we stood next to the bookshelves is still emblazoned in my mind.

Looking back on that time in my life, I'm surprised by my apparent need to be covert about seeking out information about sex. My parents, after all, are experienced sex educators. Never had they given me the impression that sex was something wrong or something to be ashamed about. But feeling like it is, is also perfectly natural. It's built into the very structure of our society. There is no point in wondering *why* we feel that way; it's more important to choose fun ways to view sex. Being willing to talk about sex and confront what it is we want is integral to having a good sex life.

It's this stigma about talking about sex that often prevents us from having safe sex. People would rather have unsafe experiences than be deliberate and talk about them.

Contrary to popular belief, safe sex is actually fun sex. I used to mentally gripe about the awkwardness of condoms, or how weird it would seem to ask a potential partner to use a latex barrier, but I eventually realized that when I'm having protected sex, I'm having more fun because I don't have to think about all those things I usually worry about if I was having a less deliberate encounter. Because trust me, I would worry about all sorts of stuff if I weren't being safe. All kinds of questions would come up: does he have anything I might get? Has he told me the truth about his past experiences? Am I putting my friend at risk right now? I realized that when I take the proper steps to use barriers, I am a lot more relaxed and I can focus on the actual point of the experience: my pleasure.

As I was growing up, my family talked to me about how to have safe sex and they readily gave me the means to do so. They established early on that I could ask them anything I could think of about sex, so I knew that I could go to them with any questions. When I actually began to have sensual experiences, they didn't tell me what to do or not do. Instead, they explained to me how to be safe. I knew about latex gloves and condoms and what kinds of lubricants are safe to use long before I actually began having sex. Studies have shown that students who have had youth sex education will not begin having sex earlier than people who have not, as is sometimes argued. Just the opposite has been demonstrated: providing youth with information about birth control was associated with positive sexual behavior as well as a delay in the beginning of sexual activity.[1]

What's this "safe sex" thing all about? Many sex education teachers have begun calling it "safer sex" because there is no such thing as completely safe, no-chance-of-contamination-you're-in-a-bubble sexual contact. Sex with another person means that there are bodies functioning in a small area together, so there is some risk no matter what. Ultimately, masturbation is the safest form of sex. But when you are ready to include another person in your experience, you can do what it takes to have those experiences be as fun and as risk-free as possible. To do so, you'll require a few tools and some good communication in order to have this happen.

It can feel difficult or even intimidating to talk to a partner about safe sex. Most of the media we are exposed to about sex does *not* include safety. In fact, a recent study concluded that 98 percent of films that include sexual acts do not include any references to contraception and most show these activities taking place between newly acquainted partners.[2] Porn and mainstream movies almost never pause to grab a pair of latex gloves before fingering or ask a partner to put on a condom or dental dam before segueing into oral sex. But with the vast potential for contracting an STI, it's important to value your health and wellness first.

So, start talking. Before I begin to get intimate with a new person, I lay out that I have safe sex practices that are important to me and, depending on what kind of activity it is that I want to do, I'll communicate the latex barriers that are required companions for that experience. It's important to tell your partner exactly what you want for several reasons. For one, they're not mind readers; they may know that you want to use condoms and also want to use them themselves, or they might not. And secondly, each person enters into a sexual experience with their own history and their own way of doing things. They might also be fans and practitioners of safe sex, or they may never have even heard of a dental dam; you'll never know until you start the conversation.

Communicating clearly and confidently is important. First, decide exactly what you want and what your goals are regarding a sexual encounter. Ask yourself: is having safe sex important to you? If your answer is "yes," proceed with that viewpoint and have that desire as non-negotiable, regardless of your partner's response. They may think using a latex barrier is "weird" or "awkward," but if you value it, they will as well. And if they don't, they're probably not worth having sex with.

Secondly, make your latex barriers readily available and use them enthusiastically. The more comfortable you are with using them, the easier the experience will be. Educate yourself about the products and practices that are right for you. This chapter contains a brief overview of the types of protection that are available and how to use them. There are many enthusiastic and brilliant educators on YouTube and other sites which contain well-researched and well-presented information on having safe sex (you can take a look at the Resources chapter of this book for URLs).

And lastly, don't buy the bullshit! You can feel plenty through a latex barrier. Try using two gloves and then removing one and see how much you can feel.* I have had experiences while having sex where I decided to stop and make sure the condom was still on because the sensation I felt was so rich and direct, I thought the condom had come off. In addition to this, using latex and lubricant can actually make the experience even better because of the smoother texture and how well everything moves (and doesn't dry out) with lube.[3] Your viewpoint on safe sex directly affects the experience that you create.

This isn't a subject to approach lightly. Anyone who has been sexually active in any sense can get an STI. According to Heather Corinna's work, *S.E.X.*, one person in every four will contract an STI and young people are the group with the highest rates of STIs.[4] If you still aren't convinced that safer sex is worth the investment, consider the fact that those with vulvas are more likely to get an STI than those with penises, since the vagina, cervix, and rectum are more easily infected due to micro-abrasions, which are similar to tiny cracks along the surfaces of these areas.[5] We are all vulnerable to infection, so it simply makes sense to take steps to protect ourselves and the people we interact with in sexual or sensual situations.

Having safer sex is comprised of three main elements: using latex barriers effectively, STI screenings, and lifestyle choices. For the remainder of this chapter, I'll describe some common latex barriers and how to use them, as well as a brief overview of the wonderful world of lubricants. Annual STI screenings and sexual health exams from a health provider are key in maintaining your own sexual health, as well as the health of people that you come into contact with.

---

* While in this example I've suggested using two layers of latex gloves as a way to establish how much can be felt through one layer of protection, it is important to note that you should *not* use two condoms at once at any point. You're actually decreasing the efficacy of your protection if you do that, because the friction between the two condoms increases the risk of them ripping or tearing. The same goes for using an inner condom and an outer condom at the same time (again, friction is created between the two layers of latex).

More frequent STI testing is necessary with new partners or if you have multiple partners. There are also different choices you can make for yourself in terms of limiting your high-risk activities, like not having unprotected intercourse, limiting any exposure to blood, and also ensuring that any of your body modifications (like piercings and tattoos) are done at a clean facility with sterile equipment.[6]

There are many reliable options for having safer sex. Condoms, gloves, dental dams, and finger cots are all available online. What follows is a brief overview of standard forms of latex barriers for safer sex.

Latex Barriers
Outer Condoms

Condoms are readily available at drug stores, grocery stores, places which provide health services (Planned Parenthood will give you a bag for free!), or online. Do a little research to find out which kind of condom will work best for you. They come in all shapes, sizes and flavors: you can get latex or non-latex, scented and flavored, textured and ribbed, lubricated or not. Also, remember to find a lubricant that will work with condoms; oil-based lubricant is not compatible with latex condoms. (Oil of *any kind* breaks down the latex and causes breakage. This includes but is not limited to: coconut oil or any cooking/body oil, lotions, and Vaseline/petroleum-based products.) Make sure that you acquire condoms which are of good quality, are not expired, and have been stored properly before use. (If they have been stored at a high or very cold temperature they can become brittle and less effective. Similarly, do not store condoms in a wallet or other location where they encounter prolonged friction, as the pressure of that friction can weaken the latex, potentially causing a breakage.)[7]

There are a few must-do's when it comes to using a condom effectively:

Use a condom for all direct genital contact. In fact, go ahead and put that condom on as soon as you're about to touch a penis, or use your penis to touch anyone else. When opening the package, be careful to avoid damaging the condom. You may think that opening a condom with your teeth looks sexier, but truly it doesn't. Scoot the condom to the side of the packaging before you tear it open. Before unrolling the condom, ensure that the condom is positioned correctly to actually let it unroll. When rolling the condom on, pinch the tip of the condom to leave room for ejaculate that may or may not occur. Use latex-safe (water-based is the best option, as mentioned) lubricant with your condoms and add more whenever you feel like it; lube is good and should be used generously! Ample lubrication will only make things better for both parties involved and will increase the efficacy of the barrier by preventing breakage. And pay attention to the after part: hold the base of the condom-clad cock before withdrawing at the end of the sex act and withdraw immediately after ejaculation. If you stay put, it's likely that ejaculate will seep out, which would defeat the purpose of using a barrier. As with all barriers, dispose of the condom after use.[8]

Gloves

Gloves are available at drug stores or online. Find a glove that is fitted (it will have a designated size, usually small, medium, or large) rather than a one-size-fits-all glove. Pro tip: a snugger fit will allow for more precision and dexterity. Latex and nitrile gloves usually provide a closer fit than polyurethane, for example. Using lubricant (again, water-based!) is an excellent idea, as gloves tend to get caught on body hair.

Gloves are easy and effective to use. Gloves protect against the transmission of bodily fluids through microscopic abrasions on the fingers and hands, which could transmit STIs. And besides that, they can actually make manual-genital contact feel better than ungloved contact, because your hands and fingers become smoother and you don't have to worry about the cleanliness of your hands. Once you have a glove on, be aware of what you touch. Touching your face, any of your own mucous membranes, or random surfaces nearby will compromise the cleanliness of the gloves. Also, if you're going to touch both the vaginal and anal areas, be careful to not cross-touch. Anal bacteria do not do well with the vagina and some nasty infections await if you're not careful.

I use latex gloves for "DO dates," during which the person DOing touches the DOee's genitals directly. This is a safe form of sex as the point of contact is between the hands and the vulva or genital area, and, by wearing a pair of gloves, there is no chance of fluid transmission (unless a non-water based lubricant is used or the gloves are compromised).

Dental Dams

A dental dam is a thin rectangle of latex or nitrile, usually six inches across, which can be used as a barrier method. Simply lay the dam over the genital area to be orally stimulated (either vulva or anus) and hold in place with your hands during the experience. In order to keep track of which side is for placing against the genital area and which is for oral contact, simply write a non-reversible letter or word on one side. Pairing a dental dam with gloves will allow for maximum protection as well as maximum ways to stimulate your partner. Also, don't forget: no swapping areas (i.e. moving from butt to vulva, or vise-versa). Instead, simply acquire a new dam and gloves before moving to the new area.

Dental dams can be a little tricky to find in brick and mortar stores but can readily be found online. Alternatively, cutting open a condom longways or cutting open a latex glove lengthwise are viable alternatives.[9] Although not FDA approved, plastic wrap (non-microwavable Saran and Cling Wrap) is also a good and accessible alternative to dental dams. This method has been approved by Planned Parenthood and the Centers for Disease Control.[10]

Inside Condoms

These are available online or at a health care provider. Inside condoms (also called "female condoms") are non-latex and are inserted inside the vaginal or anal canal and can be put in place hours before sex, which is one reason that people like to use them. They are shaped like a tube with a plastic or foam ring at the closed end which fits inside the canal. Inner condoms come in a variety of sizes, so if you are interested in using one, make sure to research the sizes available to ensure proper fit (this is of particular importance post-partum). Also, since the person with the vagina or anus gets to wear it, they get to be the one completely in charge of their own protection.

• • • • • •

That brings up an important point to note: who is responsible for ensuring that you're using protection during sex?

You are. Yep, only you. If it's what you want, you can't leave it up to the other person to take care of it. Not being adequately prepared is no excuse for having an unsafe encounter. So, set yourself up to succeed! If you're thinking about maybe one day having penis-in-vagina or anal sexual contact, go ahead and pick up some condoms. The next time you have a visit to your health provider, you may be able to request a bag of condoms, free of charge! Find out what size latex (or latex alternative) gloves fit you and have a box on hand. Take the samples offered by your healthcare provider and create a stockpile for yourself, so that when you are ready to begin having sexual contact, you won't be limited or, worse yet, put yourself in a position to compromise. You can even set up a drawer or basket in your room, a bathroom, or any area where there is space, that contains latex barriers, lubricants, and feminine hygiene supplies, whether or not you plan on using them immediately, because it makes them accessible and normalizes sexual health.

If you're already sexually active, make sure that your safer sex supplies include everything you want so that you can have the experiences you want to have, safely and without restriction: gloves, condoms, dams, the works! Keep them nearby in a bedside drawer, or somewhere within reach. There is no need to ever compromise with your safer sex practices, so set yourself up to have as much fun as possible.

So, why all this emphasis on safer sex? Well, because of STIs, of course!

Sexually transmitted infections, or STIs, include a range of health issues that are passed from person to person via sexual contact and/or swapping of bodily fluids. The main bodily fluids that transmit STIs are cervical mucus, semen, and blood. Some STIs can be transmitted through breast milk and saliva, as well. Some STIs are treatable, while others are not.

Please refer to the Resources chapter for a comprehensive list of STIs, causes of infection, and more specifics on prevention. I highly recommend consulting a physician regarding diagnosis and treatment. The intention of this book is purely educational and is in no way a substitute for consulting a medical professional. Planned Parenthood will provide information and care at a sliding scale (often without cost) and is completely confidential. You do not need parental permission to use the services of Planned Parenthood and in most states, your information is completely confidential. The Resources chapter also contains URLs of online resources for finding out the laws concerning minor's rights in your state.

Lubricant

No sex education book would be complete without information on and suggestions for lubricants. Lube is a key part of having pleasurable, fun sex. Most sexual contact, whether with yourself or another person, involves a degree of friction or rubbing in some way or another, and while our bodies produce a degree of natural lubrication, that usually won't last long or may not be present at all. Simply put: lubricants increase pleasure. While there is some stigma attached to using lubricant, know that the majority of people have used lubricant and mainly do so because it adds to the pleasure of the experience.[11]

For use with condoms, a small amount (a couple of drops) can be placed inside the condom as well as applied to the outside of the condom after it is in place. For use with a dental dam, apply the lubricant to the genital area prior to applying the dam. For use with gloves, apply to fingertips after the gloves are in place and then also onto the person's genitals.

There has been an enormous number of lubricants appearing on the market within the past couple of decades and I encourage you to do your own research as to what lubricant works best for you. In general, using a lubricant that is safe for use with latex (the label will usually specify whether or not it is right on the bottle) and has fewer ingredients is better. Be aware of any allergies you may have when making your decision. If you're having trouble deciding, many companies offer sample packs so that you can try out multiple types.[12]

There are three main types of lubricant available:

- Water Based: Safe to use with any latex barrier and is generally safe for internal use. Since it is water based and evaporates, you may have to reapply during use.

- Oil Based: This variety of lubricant is not compatible for use with latex barriers. Use an oil-based lubricant for solo-sex only. It is not safe for internal use, but since it does not evaporate, a little goes a long way and does not need to be reapplied.
- Silicone: Silicone-based lubricant is not safe for use with silicone toys (or any silicone products, for that matter), but it is compatible with latex barriers. This kind of lube tends to stay on the skin longer, even under water, which is why some people prefer this variety of lube. Must be washed off with warm, soapy water.

If you have any concern with lube making it onto your bedding, use a towel underneath yourself to easily catch any excess.

Natural Lubrication

Speaking of lubricant, let's take a moment to talk about the natural lubrication that our bodies produce. It can be a challenge to find out any information about what comes out of a vulva that's not the scary-bad stuff: it's usually warnings about what *not* to find in your panties, instead of what to expect when everything is healthy. This leaves a lot of unanswered questions for people who want to know what to expect. Usually male ejaculation is what is stressed in sex ed classes, but here's the good news: almost everybody gets to experience the joy of ejaculate, it just looks different in terms of amount, quantity, and substance depending on the body.

Both people with vaginas and people with penises will begin to experience a form of ejaculate which begins after puberty starts.[13] This is a perfectly normal part of growing up and maturing; it may be something you notice that develops gradually. Discharge also occurs, which is another natural aspect of how a vulva functions.[14]

I first found out that anything was produced "down there" when I was pretty little. My mom included it in one of our first conversations about masturbation. It came out of an observation that I made about my own body, that some sort of liquid was being produced that felt slippery. She let me know that it was natural and simply something that came with that part of my body.

Keep in mind that feeling wetness or natural discharge doesn't necessarily have anything to do with sex. It's a natural state and can occur for any number of reasons. Along those same lines, ejaculation and orgasm are not synonymous. Orgasm can happen without ejaculation, and vice versa.[15] Ejaculate and natural discharge can occur for all sorts of reasons. A few I've experienced are: feeling good, a burst of happiness for any number of reasons, seeing a person I like or feel good about, going on a run or any kind of exercise, dancing, gardening, cooking dinner, watching Netflix in bed, being alone except for a bowl of ice cream resting on my chest, reading a good book, reading the newspaper, changing my clothes. . . . You see, it's a pretty long list.

Vaginas are meant to be moist; the what, when, how, and why of natural lubrication varies wildly, but overall, they're wet. And that's a good thing. The vagina (we're talking about the internal part of female reproductive anatomy here) is like a self-cleaning oven. There are lots of good bacteria inside the vagina which help to keep everything clean, keep the pH balanced, and maintain overall vaginal health.[16]

Although vaginas and penises both naturally produce a form of lubrication, I still highly recommend using another form of lubrication, like a water-based lube, for any touching or sensual activities that may include friction of any kind. While the lubrication our bodies produces is fun and feels good, it also may or may not be present depending on the situation. An artificial lube will ensure that an activity, whether that's masturbation, a self-exam, or another intimate activity *feels as good as possible.*

· · · · · ·

Being aware of what your natural discharge and ejaculate typically look and feel like is an important part of keeping track of your health.

Discharge and ejaculate from a vulva can look pretty similar: it is typically thin in consistency and ranges from whitish to clear, but can also become quite thick and tend toward yellowish in color.[17] Ejaculate that comes out of a penis, also called semen, contains sperm (along with other fluids related to keeping sperm alive), and is usually within the range of milky and whitish to translucent, but can have yellowish coloration as well.[18] Pre-ejaculate, which can happen during arousal, can also contain sperm and is usually thin in consistency and clear.[19]

In general, it is recommended to talk to your doctor if you begin to experience or notice any intense or very strong odor (especially akin to fish and/or metal), anything green/yellow/streaked with blood (or blood of any kind, for those with a penis), or burning and itching in your genitals. Any pain with urination or ejaculation should be discussed with a medical professional as well.

Before we close this chapter, I have one last thing to say about vulvas. A vulva should smell, feel, taste, look, and be just like a vulva. That's it. That's all its gotta do. How a vagina and vulva looks/feels/smells, etcetera, varies *hugely*, whether in shape, size, labia length, clitoral size, pubic hair color/texture/length, or basically any aspect you can think of about a pussy, it looks different on someone else. What does a pussy *not* have to be? Violets. Or roses. Or "sweet breeze." Or "garden flora." Or any of that. Perfumed and deodorizing menstrual products, douching, and products whose sole function is to deodorize and/or perfume the vagina are not only unnecessary, but potentially harmful because artificial scents and perfumes can cause irritation and allergic reactions.[20]

Douching is a process in which a product is used to flush the vagina (the internal part of female genitalia). However, this process can change the pH of your vagina and interfere with your body's natural ability to clean itself and maintain a healthy balance. In fact, douching actually *increases* your chance of getting Pelvic Inflammatory Disease (PID) and may also increase odors and discharge due to the irritation douching causes. Washing your genital area with warm water and gentle soap is sufficient for taking care of your body.[21]

If the aforementioned products are something that you would like to use because it feels more comfortable to you, that is your choice and entirely up to you. But let me just be the voice in your ear that says, "Let your pussy smell and be just like a pussy: it's perfect the way it is."

Part 3

Communication

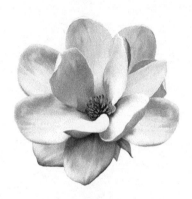

Chapter 9

DOUBLE "C's"– COMMUNICATION AND CONSENT

Communication

One evening, we ran through the living room, round and round, until we were so dizzy we would momentarily collapse in laughter before nearly instantly leaping up to resume the chase. Adults sprung aside as my sister and I tore through the house, half-naked and reckless. Darting around furniture, I leapt toward her and was caught, mid-lunge, by the upholstered arm of our living room couch. I was suddenly stopped as a searing pain ripped through my chest. Tears instantly burst from my eyes and I looked down to assess the damage: a large red swath of angry, raised flesh. I had rug burn on my nipple.

At eight, I loved to run around with no shirt on. I felt free to be as naked as I pleased. I loved to dress "like a boy" and volunteered to play the boy parts in our various plays and make-believe games. I wanted to climb trees, lay in the dirt, stay outside late, and never brush my long, brown hair. But now my nipple hurt in a way I'd never experienced. It was like a searing from the inside—this was beyond the pain of a little scrape on the knee. There was a throbbing, deeper discomfort that I couldn't simply get my Mom to blow on and make go away. My dad held me against him as I recovered and then he told me he knew exactly how I felt, that when he was a boy at the start of puberty, he remembered the particular pain and discomfort that began to grow in his own chest, and the acute tenderness of his nipples. I realized that I was getting boobs; that's what that other, more acute sensation was.

It wasn't until I was much older that I realized how novel it was that I first learned about my breasts from my dad. There seems to be a huge divide between what we can talk about with whom and a lot of it appears to be divided by our social gender roles. There's "mother-daughter time" and "father-son time," but there are prejudices about what you can talk about with whom, and of course, those certain topics people believe you can *never* talk to anyone else about.

Most people I know are surprised to hear that I talk to my parents about my sex life at all. They mostly seem to be a bit horrified at the prospect of opening up that kind of conversation with their own parents. Everyone has a different relationship with their parents or guardians, and I know that what I experienced is not possible for everyone. I also know that the guidance and direction I got from my parents and the other adults who raised me was invaluable and I would not be the person I am today without their training and communication.

Which brings me to my point: training to communicate. We can train ourselves to communicate well, just like we train for a sport or a spelling bee. The people who raised me trained me through the way they communicated with me, that is, they talked to me how they wanted to be talked to. They told me the truth. They spoke to me clearly and concisely and treated me like a totally adequate human being regardless of my age, level of education, or how I might have been behaving.

I am often asked how to get conversation started, either from the parent/guardian or youth perspective. From my perspective, the most important thing is that these conversations happen at all, regardless of how scary, challenging, or awkward they may seem. Recently, I was asked about my viewpoint on the "toxic sex environment" of college campuses. When we can casually throw around terms like "toxic" in regard to sex, amidst this burgeoning conversation around rape culture, we know that we must make different choices.

There is an enormous disconnect between how we treat young people and how we expect them to act. Until a person turns eighteen, it's not OK to talk openly with them about sex. We can't show direct pictures of female genitalia, or any pubic hair at all, because it's "immodest." We can't tell little girls the names of all their body parts (like vulva and labia) because it's "inappropriate." But then once a person is a full-grown adult, we expect them to make positive, educated decisions around sex immediately.

So yes, it can certainly be difficult to talk to your parent or your child about sex. But in the bigger picture, we have to make different choices and open up the conversation. We can create larger change through making new, pleasure-oriented choices on a micro scale. We cannot change other people's behavior, but we can change ours. By deliberately making choices each day to improve your own life and those of your friends, you are changing the world.

It starts with one conversation. And since conversing about pleasure, sensuality, or anything that we have emotional charge attached to can be challenging, I've found it helpful to break down what successful communication is into the individual components that make it work.

First, pick the person you want to communicate with and put your attention on them before you even start talking. Consider the other person: Are they ready to have this conversation? Or, are they busy making a smoothie? Putting your attention on the other person and noticing them is the first step. Next, decide what you want in this conversation, your *intent* for communicating. Think about what your objective for communicating is or what goals you have with the person. Whether they are a relative, your friend from high school, or someone you just met, you can use your intention to have what you want from a conversation. Attention and intention are the first steps of clear communication.

Once you have figured out what you want to say, introduce your topic to them. This is called "safe porting,"* which is when you tell someone what you're going to do before you do it. (Pro tip: this is a particularly useful tool in DOing and in any sensual experience.) You can ask if they'd like to talk to you about something more personal or ask if it's OK if you ask them about a more intimate topic than usual. If you get a person's agreement first, you will have a much greater rate of success in your communications. Broaching the topic before you dive right into it ensures that the person you want to talk with is receptive.

---

* Please see the Resources section at the end of this book for a further explanation of the term "safe port."

Next, ask your question, or describe your experience with as little emotion as you can. Reporting about your experience in a way that's not dramatic or full of emotion is a more effective way of having people hear you. Taking a moment to gather your thoughts about what you really want to say, whether it's negative or positive, will help you communicate more clearly. Usually I call this being neutral or not having "charge." Charge is any value judgment that you make on a situation, whether it's negative or positive.

Those are the four most important steps to successful communication. Keep in mind that ultimately, it only takes one person to be responsible for a communication. A lot of people seem to think that communication is some kind of magic. That you put these words out there randomly and that people say something back, and however it goes is really fifty-fifty; it could go well or go poorly, and they have no control over the outcome. However, there is another way which guarantees success every time, and that's through using the tools that I described. It only takes one person to be responsible for a communication; it's not dependent on the other person at all. That is great news for anyone who wants to start talking to the important people in their life and build better relationships with them.

My mom is a person in my life whom I've had a lot of my most meaningful life-changing conversations with. She's been the main person I've turned to when I wanted something new, I wanted a change, or I was going to make a major life decision of any kind. Over a decade ago, she was the person I sought out to speak with when I was considering having intercourse for the first time.

While my Mom drove me home from soccer practice one evening, I told her that I wanted to have sex for the first time. It was late fall and the sky was cool gray, announcing the upcoming winter. The river had a steely-black look that often happens around dusk when it's near freezing. As we whizzed by on curvy roads, I could see the bare oak trees and red willows curling up from along the river bank. I had been sitting on my announcement for several miles, contemplating saying anything at all.

I was fifteen then and had decided that it was time. I'd been seeing a boy from my soccer team for several months and had been thoroughly enjoying kissing him. We'd kiss for hours at a time with big, enthusiastic mouths. I once kissed him for so long that I got leg cramps from sitting in a bizarre, non-ergonomic position while leaning against a flat slab of stone. We spent a lot more time kissing than we did talking, but that didn't matter much at the time. I figured he was a good one to do it with since I'd known him for a while and he seemed like a good guy.

As I deliberated raising this subject, my stomach had a familiar warm and tightly swirling sensation that I get when I have a lot of emotions attached to what I want to say. I knew that I wasn't going to go through with the whole sex thing without telling her first, so I figured I'd just go for it. Finally, I blurted it out in a fit of word-vomit: "I'm going to have sex with him." I figured that if I said, "I am" instead of "I'm thinking about" or even "I want to," that she'd take me more seriously and think I was inflexible on the matter. I expected a reaction, an argument. She, however, was unfazed and continued watching the road in front of her, driving swiftly and calmly as each wide curve unfolded. Then, asking in a straightforward tone after a nearly imperceptible pause, "Are you sure that you want to do that?" Gazing at her profile, with her short wavy hair and fair skin, I was momentarily dumbstruck. I now had to consider bigger questions than I'd been willing to look at so far, namely: Am I sure? Why him? Why now?

The conversation continued from there. She asked me the questions that I was suddenly confronting and she gave me the space to answer them. My mom has always let me say what I have to say without trying to fix me. By simply asking questions and letting me answer them, she facilitated my realization that fucking this guy was not, in fact, what I wanted after all. Looking back on the choices that I eventually made in regard to having sexual encounters, I am grateful for that moment of pause, for that quiet along the curves of the river where my mom put her attention on me and viewed me without value in a circumstance of immense charge.

Consent

Now that we have some of the fundamentals of communication in place, we can explore the other "C" of this chapter: consent.

Since I was homeschooled until the age of sixteen when I started college, I had a relatively insulated experience growing up, interrupted only by the twenty adults I lived with, my sister, soccer and swim practice, and the people that were constantly streaming in and out of our property to take courses to expand their ideas of sensuality and communication (so perhaps not that insulated, after all). There were a few things that surprised me when I started functioning in a more "public" environment like the local city college.

One of these ideas was "consent."

I'd never heard people use this word the way I started to hear it, especially in the Human Sexuality course I took to fulfill a general education requirement, but certainly not limited to that corner of my world. I started to see it in articles online and heard it discussed amongst my peers, especially once I started university and began to learn more about the special culture of a college campus, complete with Greek life and half the student population housed in on-campus dormitories. Now, many years post-graduation, I see the word more than ever in the midst of our collective #MeToo conversation where thousands of women, men, and gender non-binary people have stood up to acknowledge when they did *not* give consent. This word has entered new heights of usage as we try to educate people about how, and why, to talk to each other and communicate when and if they want to physically interact in particular ways.

And still, this word is unfamiliar to me.

It's not a word I was raised with, which is surprising because my parents are some of the most sex-positive and communicative people I've ever met. So, when I looked back over my life and my upbringing, I looked for an answer as to why I wasn't raised with this concept.

I was taught to ask for what I wanted, whether it was for a sugary dessert or a ride to town. Since we lived forty-five minutes from the next town and on a sugar-restricted diet, I grew up asking for lots of things. On top of that, I had a sister close in age to me and we were also taught to always, *always* look out for each other. So, if I was given something, I had to figure out a way to get one for her too, or to split mine to share with her, because I knew she'd do the same for me. All of this required constant communication on all our parts and had the effect of training me very early on to speak up and ask for what I wanted.

Later on, when I learned about sex, I learned about it from the perspective of having what I wanted, nothing else. The dialogue was always "when you want to . . ." and "when you decide . . . ," never, "if you find the right person . . ." or "when you're eighteen . . ." The responsibility was always in my court, just like all the other aspects of my life.

When I had the first sexual encounter with my first partner, it was all through communication. I asked him to have a DO date and in that instance I asked him to stroke my clitoris with his fingertip. Of course, I was blushing like mad and his eyes were so squinted from his huge smile that I could barely see them directly, but the words came out and we got on the bed. Throughout the experience, he asked me if I wanted specific changes and I'd answer "yes" or "no" or ask him for a change myself, which meant we both knew the whole time what we were both experiencing and what we each wanted.

When I think back on that experience, I realize how these fundamental ideas of consent, asking if the person would like to have sex, and if so, checking in during the experience to ensure all parties are still in agreement, was built into my life. And not just my sex life, but through the fundamental way in which we ran our household, how we planted the garden, and even how we decided who would drive to town. My community's teaching business is called "The Welcomed Consensus," as in, welcoming agreement by all parties. They only make decisions when every single person in the group is a "yes," or in agreement with what is being decided upon or the direction of the group. As a result, we've had house meetings that went on for, I kid you not, *hours* because people were not in agreement about how we were going to plant our summer garden. It may seem tedious or inefficient to spend that much time discussing the finer points of using a tractor or building a trellis, but if you've ever built something with a person *not* in agreement with what's happening, you'll know it's worth the investment.

One of the basic agreements of our community is the "one no vote" rule, which works exactly how it sounds. I've mentioned "house meetings" a few times, which are when the whole household gets together for a meeting which can last from fifteen minutes to several hours and can cover any range of topics from logistics regarding an upcoming event, a new person joining the community, or specific aspects of each person's day or daily experience; there's a huge range. A house meeting is a place where a vote might take place, but frankly we almost never vote because it is usually clear without it whether or not we're all in agreement with each other.

I was six the first time I remember us all voting on something. We were having a house meeting so all of us were gathered in the living room and together formed a ring that outlined the entire room. Sophia and I didn't always go to the meetings and sometimes when we did, it was mainly so we could listen in from the comfort of our Mom's lap or spooned up against our Dad's side. In this particular meeting, we each had our own seat, which was a sign of its gravity. Someone was on the brink of leaving; the details are hazy, but I remember the person was on the outs with the whole group. Everyone wanted this person out of there and we were taking it to a vote, all in favor of the person leaving were to raise their hands. (As an aside, this was an extremely rare circumstance; in the twenty-two years since I've been living there nothing like this has occurred again—people either leave or decide to stay, there is almost never a need for voting.)

The heat in the room still sticks with me. People were in agreement with this person packing up and shipping out. I raised my hand along with everyone else—all except Sophia, that is. I looked to my right and saw her hands firmly at her sides and a set expression on her face. Quickly, all the adults turned and realized there was dissent and the vote broke up. So-and-So got to stay, and apparently, they ended up living with us for several more months. I felt taken aback by her choice. She'd gone against that whole group and stood up for what she thought was right. I knew even then that we collectively held the viewpoint that anyone who wanted could live with us, and she'd been the one to stick to that viewpoint, no matter what her own parents thought, no matter that she was on average at least twenty-five years younger than everyone there.

That was a moment when I realized the weight of my own voice. That could just as easily have been my hand that swayed the whole group. That's what our parents and our style of living taught us: that our voices mattered. There was a way they managed to treat my sister and me like adults without ever stopping being our parents. No, we couldn't eat as much candy as we wanted to, stay up all night jumping on our beds, or play in the street, but we could stand shoulder to shoulder with the rest of the group and make decisions. Valuing the importance of our own voice and choices is a key aspect of consent itself.

What is consent?

Consent is when the people participating in a sexual act are in agreement with what is happening. Consent is ongoing; just because a person agreed at the beginning of the experience doesn't mean that they can't change their mind at *any* point. Silence does not mean consent; nothing but a verbal "yes" means consent. Any sexual contact without agreement is sexual assault or rape. Sexual contact can include, but is not limited to, penetration, oral sex, and genital touching.

This subject is being discussed more and more openly, from middle schools to college campuses. The are many excellent resources to read more online: RAAIN (Rape, Abuse & Incest National Network),[1] Planned Parenthood,[2] and Heather Corinna's website "Scarleteen,"[3] all contain more information about aspects of consent and information about how consent and sexual assault laws vary depending on the US state or country. Below is a guide compiled from the previously named sources to get a conversation started about what consent means.

Consent is . . . [4]

Deliberate, as it's saying yes to one sexual act which does not automatically mean "yes" for other acts. Each part of a sensual encounter is independent from another (i.e. just because you say yes to holding hands doesn't mean you'll get into bed with them. Just because you agreed to oral sex doesn't mean you've also agreed to penetrative sex.).

Given *without pressure* (from peers, socially, or otherwise) and without the influence of alcohol or drugs.

Withdrawn at any point before or during the sexual encounter, without need for explanation, regardless of whether or not you've done it before or if you just met the person.

Communicated fully. You can only consent to something if all the information is on the table. For example, if a person says they will use birth control, but then does not, that is *not* consent.

What you *want*: enthusiastic sex is the best kind of sexual contact to have; it's sex without expectation or feelings of obligation.

• • • • • •

Communication is a vital aspect of any consensual experience. But we're not usually taught to communicate about sex. Directly asking if a person wants to have sex is usually thought of as awkward or too blunt and speaking during sex is nearly unheard of. However, those are cultural taboos and personal limitations, both of which are simply points of view and are subject to change depending on what your goals are. Communication is inherent to sex itself and there are many ways to communicate before, during, and after a sensual act. And, in my experience, the best sex is talked-about sex.

Talking before, during, and after adds to a sensual experience immensely and is a good way to check in and ensure all parties involved are happy with the experience they're having. By communicating your own enjoyment (which could mean explicitly describing a particular aspect that you're enjoying), you're letting the other person know that the experience is good for you and that you're both succeeding. Verbally stating your own enjoyment and asking your partner about their experience can be a turn on and add even more fun. Further, by communicating yourself, you then create an opportunity for the other person to acknowledge how they feel and if they would like any changes.

If talking about sex seems too difficult, you may not be ready to have it. A sign of knowing what you want is an ability to articulate it. Talking about what you want, whether that's a spooning session on the couch or a sloppy make-out session in the bathroom, can feel confrontational because it *is*: you're confronting what you want. By starting a conversation, you get an opportunity to envision and create the experience you want to have, which can shift and grow through the conversation itself. If this feels impossible, I suggest taking some time for yourself to consider what your wants and goals are. Journaling or talking with someone you're close with can be good ways to air considerations before you're ready to actually have the experiences.

One of the underlying viewpoints behind people not wanting to ask if another person would like to have sex is based on the fear that they will say no. In my opinion, that's an even better reason to ask: if the other person is at all reluctant or less than enthusiastic, it won't be a fun sensual experience!

It's safest to use actual words when engaging in a sensual experience. Many people may prefer nonverbal communication or body language, which can certainly be successful. But if you're new to sensual engagements, are with a new partner, have difficulty reading body language, or are feeling any doubt about what's going on, definitely use verbal communication. No matter how many times you've had sex or how many times you and your partner have had sex, you still must have agreement about the encounter.

There are many ways to go about this. Some ideas are to frame a request with "may I . . ." or "I'm interested in [blank], are you interested in that?" Both of these forms of questions are open-ended and don't put pressure on the person being asked the question. Being open and flexible with your intention and the words you choose leaves room in the conversation for the other person to agree, decline, or make a new offer.

• • • • • •

Jaclyn Friedman, co-editor of *Yes Means Yes*, has a perfect explanation of consent and sex:

> Sexual consent isn't like a lightswitch, which can be either "on," or "off." It's not like there's this one thing called "sex" you can consent to anyhow. "Sex" is an evolving series of actions and interactions. You have to have the enthusiastic consent of your partner for all of them. And even if you have your partner's consent for a particular activity, you have to be prepared for it to change. Consent isn't a question. It's a state. If, instead of lovers, the two of you were synchronized swimmers, consent would be the water. It's not enough to jump in, get wet and climb out—if you want to swim, you

have to be in the water continually. And if you want to have sex, you have to be continually in a state of enthusiastic consent with your partner.[5]

I love Friedman's use of synchronized swimmers as an analogy for sensual interaction with another person and how consent works in that setting and believe it's a perfect summary for the ideas explored in this chapter under the umbrella of communication. A continual state of enthusiastic consent, as she describes, is a recipe for an excellent sensual experience. Using your communication skills to ensure you and your partner are having what you want are key to ensuring a good experience for everyone involved.

Communicating what you want and ensuring the activities you are having are being enthusiastically received are fundamental aspects of communication. To take it one step further, I'd like to discuss an important aspect of successful communication, which are "specific frames."

A specific frame is when you describe a particular moment of time in detail, as if you were to pause a video and describe the relevant details of what you saw: the setting, the time of day, who is there, et cetera. Depending on the situation, you can use any (or all) of your senses to add to your specific frame. You can use specificity in many situations, including talking to other people (especially friends) and in your own writing (like in a journal).

Specific frames are useful. If you are talking to another person and you use specific frames to communicate, they have a better idea of your experience and what your life is like. This can be as simple as your daily experience. For example, if a friend asks how your day was, instead of giving a trite "fine," you can add details from some particular aspect of your day: a highlight from a meal, a fun exchange you had with another person, or a piece of music you're enjoying. You are probably already doing this in your life to some degree. Intentionally adding more specifics into your communication will add to your relationships and also be a useful tool when communicating during times of increased emotional charge, whether that's negative or positive.

Using specific frames in situations where you or the other person has more charge (by charge I mean emotional value) is very handy. If you are willing to use specific frames, you can communicate clearly. Examples of potentially charged times are during sensual experiences, during times where you or another person feels jealous, or when you're angry. But really, any situation could be a good time to increase your intention and use specific frames to succeed in your communication. Mystery only exists because of a lack of communication.

Sensual experiences are also a great time to be specific. Before you get on the bed, you can start with telling your partner what you want. It doesn't have to be set in stone, it can change, but starting the interaction by communicating what you want increases the likelihood that you'll get you want. You can start anywhere: "I'd like to have a DO date," or "Let's sit down and talk for a few minutes."

During a sensual experience, you can include your partner in what you're feeling by describing your experience in specific frames. None of us are mind readers and no matter how close you may feel to a person, there is still more for them to know about you. You can communicate anything you feel: "I have tingles in my right calf," "that pressure is perfect, it feels like a warm breeze on my skin," or "when you moved like that, it felt like a wave inside my body." Specific frames can be short. At their essence a specific frame is simply the moment the experience happened and your value judgment, or your perception. Or, they can be longer, and you can use your additional senses to provide information. More communication only adds more to the experience.

You can also communicate in specifics after the experience by telling your partner about your enjoyment. For example, you could tell them how much you enjoyed it when they started rubbing your shoulders because you felt more grounded afterward. Whatever it was that stood out to you, you can tell your partner about it.

Specifics frames are in contrast to being general. Generalities can actually create mystery because the person you're communicating with may actually have less information than when you started. Merely telling someone "that feels good" is general because they don't know exactly what it is that you're enjoying. Is it the speed? The pressure? Is it the sensation of the soft sheets against your skin? "It" could be anything!

Keep in mind that general questions will also lead to general answers. A specific question is anything that can be answered with "yes" or "no." This is especially useful in sensual experiences. If you ask your partner if they'd like more pressure, for example, they can answer with a simple "yes" or "no." If they say "yes," you can increase the pressure by an increment and then ask again, perhaps they want more pressure after that. If so, their "yes" will indicate that, or their "no" will let you know that you're using the right pressure. However, if you ask someone if that's the right pressure, or even worse, if "that's good," you may or may not like the answer you get. What if it's not good? It also puts unnecessary pressure on your partner to lie or tell you that things feel good when they actually don't. Most people don't like hurting each other's feelings, so don't create situations for that in your own communications. Ask specific questions that your partner can answer "yes" or "no" to for the most fun in sensual situations.

Simply put: good communication will lead to having more fun conversations, closer relationships, and, ultimately, more fun sex. Using these specific tools will help you get more out of your conversations and you'll end up feeling closer to the people you are communicating with. And, you'll be asking for what you want and giving your partner what they want. With these practices in place, when you're not ready to do something or if things are not going your way, you'll be willing to talk about it.

Chapter 10

NUTS AND BOLTS
OF FRIENDSHIP

While writing and researching this chapter on relationships and specifically on friendships, I came across the etymology of the word "friend" which relates to some of the defining principles of friendship that are particularly relevant now, hundreds of years along into our usage of the word:

> *Freond,* the Old English source of Modern English *friend* is related to the
> Old English source of Modern English *friend*, is related to the Old English
> verb *Freon*, "to love, like, honor, set free (from slavery or confinement)."
>
> Specifically, *freond* comes from the present participle of the Germanic
> ancestor of Old English *Freon* and thus originally meant "one who loves."
>
> The Germanic root of *freond* and *Freon* is *fri w*hich meant "to like,
> love, to be friendly to."[1]

The association between friendship and liking will not be too much of a surprise to anyone because it's fairly common to think of friends as people you like. However, that the original root word for "friend" meant "one who loves" is of particular relevance. Often people will use the term "friend" fairly casually; it's the term for people who aren't related to them by blood or familial ties or for the people whom they see socially but do not engage with sexually. It also has a very wide range of uses: a friend could be someone you meet up with at a café a few times a year or someone that you've known your whole life and talk to every day. These are two very different degrees of closeness, yet the same term is used for both. But the idea of love gives the word more heft. That guy I meet up with at the café? I don't love him and he surely does not love me. This has me thinking that, perhaps, I should have another term to distinguish him from the person I do talk to every day and do, in fact, love.

Secondly, there is the history of being associated with the concept of freedom, specifically to "set free." This is an aspect of friendship that is particularly fascinating because you are not bound to your friends in any legal or genetic way. You pick each other. For whatever the reason, in whatever circumstances, all friends are chosen. You may have been put together as babies in those infamous little play dates of long ago, or maybe you bumped into each other in your middle school cafeteria. You may have liked her bangs, or his shoes, but for some reason, you picked them and they in turn picked you right back. Friendship requires choice and there is a freedom in that.

My family ingrained in me when I was a little kid that friends are important; they told me that friends are the highest form of relationship a person can have.

I was about nine years old, standing barefoot with my dad on our gravel driveway when my dad told me he was my best friend and as part of that, he would always tell me the truth. Granted, he was also my parent, so he was not going to let me screw up too badly or put myself in mortal danger; it was his biggest priority at the time to ensure that he successfully parented me in all the necessary and practical ways. However, at the same time he planted this idea in my head that he was also my friend and that friendship wasn't something to be taken lightly or casually. He said the words to me with a certain weight, a heft that hasn't left my mind.

Plus, it's something he has repeated to my sister and me so many times that it's not something we can ignore: it's emblazoned in our minds. As their children, you have some biological reasons for not viewing your parents as friends. Until you are a certain age, they are there to take care of you. They're there to keep you safe, warm, fed, and watered. To love you, tell you what's what, and point you in the right direction.

But eventually that relationship dynamic changes and there can be a time of transition. This is when you are able to take care of yourself, yet you're all still operating in the same space, whether that's in the same household, through regular Skype calls, or the occasional phone call. You're still relating but now you're both adults, which is a time when the relationship dynamic between parent/guardian and child can shift.

This is an idea I've been exploring my entire life, ever since my Dad told me he was my best friend all those years ago. Ever since then, he's demonstrated it in every conversation we've had. I haven't always liked it—I haven't always liked *him*, in fact—but it has taught me how to be a friend. And now, all grown up, I'm a friend to my Dad, too.

• • • • • •

While I've mainly focused this little monologue on parents, there are similar dynamics at play in all of our relationships: siblings, cousins, aunties, friends from kindergarten, friends from college—the list goes on.

I define a friend as a person I tell the truth to and one who tells me the truth. For the rest of this chapter I have stories that highlight different aspects of friendship.

My Sister

My sister and I were born 362 days apart, a fact we relished telling anyone we happened to come across.

Upon first meeting, no one even thinks we're related. Anyone who claims to see similarities between us immediately gets written down in the "bullshitter" column of my little black book. We look very unalike: I'm short and tend toward curvy; she's tall and lean. She has curly hair; I have thick, stick-straight hair. I have hazel eyes; she has brown. The dissimilarities go on and on. But we are close and perhaps it's the closeness that people perceive, those "bullshitters" who claim we look alike.

We're half-sisters, which I'd sometimes tell people as if to compensate for the fact that we look nothing alike. But I've realized, slowly and steadily over the years, that I do not need to explain myself. Or my sister, for that matter.

Sometimes, instead of apologizing away our relationship, we just tell them our birthdays and let them figure it out on their own: my mom actually went into labor with me on the night of Sophia's first birthday party.

This is all to say that I've always had a sister. Imagining my life without her, without another human at my side, is impossible. Until I sat down to write this, I'd never actually considered my life as a whole if Sophia had never been born. We have seamlessly and ceaselessly functioned side by side for nearly thirty years.

You may be thinking, "yawn, most sisters feel this way about one another." And I'm sure you're right. There is a bond between siblings that some are able to take full advantage of, as we have. Yet how many sisters have shared a room for their whole lives? How many have shared a *bunk bed* for most of that time?

You see, we grew up in an intentional community together. And two key aspects of our community is that we have lots of shared spaces and very few bathrooms. It's an excuse to relate and has people treat each other more nicely: how long can you really stay mad when you have to communicate well enough to take a shower while another person needs to pee and yet another has to brush their teeth? We're a close group with few limitations regarding that elusive concept of "personal space" and that's how we like it.

Sophia and I have shared a room and a bunk bed for most of our lives. When we were barely walking, we had a custom-made set of bunk beds that had rolling crib doors. Next, we had a trundle bed which didn't last long because it required one of us making our bed every single morning in order to put the underbed away for the daytime. For one sister to have to make a bed and the other not to, that's simply unfair. After that, we had a fire-engine-red metal-framed beauty that until very recently was still in use by our younger cousin. After that we had wood-framed twin beds that could either be stacked as bunk beds or separated into individuals. I was entering puberty at this time and still fondly recall the giant N*Sync, Brandy, and Spice Girls posters that covered my nook of wall and ceiling (I'd covertly kiss my boy bands and Brandy when I was in the room alone). Separating our bunks after felt like a step toward independence, a hint of adulthood. But by the time we were fifteen, we were back in bunks, but this time custom designed by a new person that joined our community.

We have a particular closeness, which may or may not have to do with our continual proximity to one another: even if we don't have to speak to one another, we are on a similar system, and we walk parallel paths through our days.

Which doesn't mean that we have always liked each other. The only person I've gotten into a fist fight with is her. We'd scratch and claw and yank at each other until one of us got hurt enough to stop the game. More frequently, we'd hurl words at each other across rooms and through closed doors, calling each other bitches, liars, and fucking assholes. The worst words we could think of.

And there were times of not talking as well. Puberty was a long stretch of silence between us. The changes we went through, her a year ahead of me, were intense and so consuming that I remember very little of relating to her. While I tended to let everyone and their momma know how I felt about my body changing and how much I wanted to get my period, Sophia went about this time very differently and very quietly. We each had our own way of doing things and eventually we reconnected after many of the hurdles of puberty were behind us.

There was a time that stands out where my sister went from covering her body at all times, including in the shower, to living in a pink polka dot bikini for the entire summer. It wasn't until I wrote this chapter that I figured out what had happened.

One summer a friend of a friend sent their young son from Belgium to our family for the summer. His parents had been childhood best friends with a woman who lives in our community, so it seemed like a fun idea to everyone involved. We were all about the same age, I was twelve and Sophia and he were about thirteen years old. His name was Leonard but we called him "Leo" the whole summer. He barely spoke a word of English and, despite years of French class, Sophia and I only had two handfuls of French between us. Although after those months together, we had at least another mouthful of French profanity ready to unleash whenever an occasion called.

Looking back on it, Leo was a sweet kid. He was rather pale and somewhat mousy-haired, but he had piercing blue eyes and a quick smile. And considering everything I put him through, he was also a terribly nice and patient person. Although I did not appreciate any of that at that time: I did not like Leo. In fact, over those months together, I grew to hate him.

There was no real reason to dislike him, besides the fact that he didn't have all the same rules that we did. Sophia and I had to keep going to school, even though it was summertime. Leo was here on vacation, so no school for him. Sophia and I had to exercise every day for at least an hour and of course, Leo had no such requirement. He didn't even have restrictions on sugar like we did, which was unbearably frustrating. Looking back on it, I am surprised by how angry I felt about it. He never said anything negative or mean-spirited toward me or anyone in my family. (How could he? None of us spoke French.) So the hostility I remember feeling seems so foreign all these years later.

I realized recently that it had to do with Sophia. Leo was the first boy we'd lived with for any length of time that either wasn't related to us or we hadn't been in diapers with. It went from just the two of us (and our troupe of adult companions) to the two of us plus a boy. A cute boy. And she liked him quite a bit, later labeling him as her first "real" crush.

One day after he'd returned to Belgium, she showed me a picture of the two of them spooned into one of those giant circle chairs that were ubiquitous in the early 2000s. Seeing the picture, their closeness and unbridled smiles, I felt a quick stab of jealousy. This was my first clue.

Before that, I'd mainly been consumed by my dislike of him. In my mind, my sister and I were a team and he was the intruder and enemy. But over those months, I saw her changing before my eyes. She shed her baggy clothes and exchanged them for a two-piece bathing suit. She began grooming herself differently as well; this was the first summer she shaved her armpits. I watched these changes and felt bewildered.

He was the first person we'd met who might come in between us. When you're two sisters growing up in the same room, sharing the same desk in your little homeschool classroom, each of you is all the other has. Of course we had many adults, many parents, and plenty of acquaintances, but we were this inseparable force. And this guy and all the energy I felt from both of us around him signaled a change. I realize now, many years later, that the part that stung was the exclusion. Suddenly she was immersed in a world that I wasn't a part of. I went from feeling like I knew everything about her, to seeing a picture of her and realizing what had transpired.

Over time, Sophia and I have realized that our relationships with others do not need to exclude one another. When we were in our later teens, my dad talked to us about how, every time we got a boyfriend we'd stop talking to him and seem to completely disappear. I didn't quite get what he was talking about at the time, as I was too wrapped up in whatever boy I had my eyes on, but in hindsight, looking back that summer with Leo and how my relationship with Sophia shifted, I began to wrap my head around it.

My sister and I were born into our relationship. I didn't choose her and she certainly didn't pick me. By reason of our positions within our beautiful community, we were able to school together, sleep in the same room, and play together our whole lives. But as we got older, we realized that friendship is different. It's a choice, every moment. Choosing to relate as friends has created one of the most valuable relationships in my life, something stronger than the definition and confines of "sisters."

My Dad

There are a lot of cultural limitations in place about the kinds of relationships we can have, particularly with those that are close to us, like our blood relatives and lovers. I mean "cultural limitations" in a general sense on purpose, because the rules for these relationships vary from culture to culture. I am speaking from the perspective of a woman raised in California from the 1990s through present day and the kind of conditioning, or rules, boundaries and restrictions, that I learned from the society I live in are different than that of people from different races, cultures, places of birth, generations, et cetera. However, some of our cultural rules are shared, like: don't have sex before marriage. That's a big one that many different religions and social structures adhere to. Even though that isn't something I believe in, it's still a part of my cultural conditioning because a) I am aware of this rule and b) I'm aware that it's a rule of other people's, as a sexually active unmarried woman, that I break.

One of the rules that we seem to hold is a set of restrictions on how we interact with our parents. Although we are supposed to love each other and treat our parents with respect, we're not supposed to tell them everything about our lives or tell them what we really think. This is a viewpoint that is spelled out to us in every teeny-bopper movie in which the teen escapes her family home to do what she'd really like to be doing, or when people experiment with drugs supposedly unbeknownst to their parent, or really any time a character avoids telling a parent something for fear of retribution. And, in a way, this makes sense. Our parents are the first people who love us and they may be the people who love us the most of anyone in our entire lives. That has a strong effect on a person and valuing what they think is natural, to the point that we'd even attempt to hide things that we don't like or feel right about in ourselves for fear of not being approved of by a parent (or guardian, or whichever title the person is who takes care of you uses).

There is also this fascinating phenomenon of exclusivity that seems to crop up alongside dating. I'm sure I'm not alone in the experience of a new person coming into my lives that I like (or have a crush on, decide to begin dating, et cetera) becoming the most important thing in the world, and having the rest of my relationships (like those with my parents or friends) become less important. My dad saw this happening right about the time my sister and I entered our teens: we'd started spending hours on the phone with people we'd only met recently, we suddenly wanted to be in town all the time to go to social events, or we'd have our attention on the person of interest when they visited and no one else. We'd go from having close, fun relationships with our dad to completely cutting him out of our lives until that object of interest became less interesting for whatever reason. Now, as an adult, I see this happening all the time: a teenager gets a boy/girl/person-friend and they disappear from their family and friend's lives, only to return months or years later, if they're lucky. But I've learned that it doesn't need to be this way; we don't actually need to exclude one another, particularly when we approach our relationships from a friendship model.

As I described earlier, my parents did their very best to teach my sister and me, and later our brothers, to be friends with each other and with them. "Friend" in this sense doesn't mean the person I hang out with the most socially or that we gossip over the latest celeb crush, but it's a person that I tell the truth to and they to me. That is a rare form of relationship and there are only a few people in my life that have that title.

My friendships with my parents look a lot of different ways and it's actually a big part of what's being explored in this entire book; after all, they raised me and they're the reason I'm sitting here, writing this thing. The stories I selected to write about my dad highlight two aspects of our relationship which are important: my willingness to talk to him and his willingness to talk to me.

Walking beside my dad on the hillside above our house, pine needles crunching underfoot and daffodils peeking up at us from around the bases of the trees, we both looked at the ground. I am not sure what we were looking for or at, but he was looking down as he walked, so I did the same. We had no real purpose to our steps, although I knew eventually we'd be making our way back to the house. Breaking the quiet between us, he asked me, "Why don't you like Celine?"

His question took me aback, not because he was off track, but because he knew at all. It's not that I thought my dislike for her was imperceptible; it was more that I hadn't confronted it myself. At the time, I was getting into a lot of arguments with people, or, more accurately, I was yelling at a lot of people, since the interactions were largely one-sided. I had a lot of energy in my body, I had just entered my teens and the daily runs, soccer practices, hours of school work, and various chores simply weren't enough to match the tornado that sometimes felt like was spinning inside me. So as another outlet, I'd take on enemies, pick fights, and wage silent wars. I once made an actual list of all the reasons why one woman, who lived in our community for years and was one of the people running the communal kitchen (and thus a sometimes-boss of me) was a terrible person. I think I actually gave her the list directly.

But I had a particular tension with Celine. I'd focused a lot of attention and negativity on her without even knowing all the reasons why. At the time she was becoming particularly close to my Dad and I believe I felt threatened by that relationship.

When he asked me the question, I had to take stock of what I was doing. Not only did I not realize that anyone else knew how I felt about her, but I had to confront that it was how I was relating to her. My dislike for her had a particular bent; it was more than just a passing annoyance like one person's tendency to ask for vegetables to be chopped *just so*.

I do not know what I told my Dad. I said a few sentences, he nodded, and the conversation ended there. I was left with my own choices.

Our relationship did not change overnight; I wasn't suddenly some kind of angelic wonderchild that adored everyone in my community (although, deep down, of course I did adore everyone; I just let other crap get in the way at times). But over time, choice by choice, Celine has become one of my closest friends. She's not a mother to me, but she's been in my life since I was six years old and she knows things about me that very few people do. From her position, she's been able to watch me grow, see the choices I've made, and offer me guidance when I was ready for it. And since she isn't my "mom" exactly, although I've often felt the intimacy of that particular shape of relationship, I could also bring things to her that I didn't want to take to my mom or dad, particularly when the subject I wished to discuss was about one of them.

All along there has been this figurative harpoon jutting out of me labeled "why don't you like Celine?" which I've periodically bumped into. Each time I feel that special pang, it's a reminder to go toward being a friend, because that direction is filled with an infinite pool of possibilities not limited by cultural conditions.

• • • • • •

The three of us sat together on the bed, speaking in a quick flow of communication. I was a bit teary but feeling more relieved as each of us spoke and aired our viewpoints on the topic. The more the two women I sat with told me about their experiences and how, for lack of a better term, "normal" my situation was, the quieter my mind felt and the more I could physically quiet down.

Moments before, I'd had one of the greatest spikes of energy in my whole life. That tiny pink line on the plastic stick of the home pregnancy kit had appeared. I knew it would, as I'd been experiencing what I'd later come to find was the evidence of pregnancy for a full six weeks. But seeing the confirmation right there in my hand, directly from my own body, I felt shock. I was supposed to have my shit together, for one. Not only did I use safe sex to a point of religion (ironic terminology aside), I even wrote about safe sex and espoused the benefits of safer sex to my friends and peers. But here I was, unexpectedly pregnant. I felt like I'd failed.

After internally screaming for a few moments, I found my closest friends and told them what was going on. We gathered in a private area to discuss the situation and generally just let me run my thoughts on the matter. We were cozily sitting together as this dramatic time in my life slowly unfolded and began turning toward resolution when my Dad walked in.

Immediately, the temperature in the room shifted. I halted, unsure of what to say next. Sensing this immediately, he quipped as he turned toward the door to leave, "Oh, this is women's stuff."

What he said was right on and I knew it straight off. That's the value judgment I'd made when he walked in and he felt it distinctly; we were discussing topics that were not in his area of expertise or any of his business. But then, I began to consider the implications of that viewpoint. Why was he not qualified? Because he doesn't have a uterus?

My dad is not just any dad. He's my best friend and the one who has always told me the truth, no matter what. No matter how big of a bitch I was being, how much of an angel, or how happy I felt. There has never been a "right time" or a "wrong time" for him to tell me the truth; he knew it was more important to talk to me and give me reality than skirt my feelings of doubt, embarrassment, or anger. He's also been teaching about human sexuality since before I was born. He's beyond experienced. Furthermore, he's been married, divorced, become a father, and been with many women who had determined for themselves when and if they'd wanted children. Suffice it to say that he was well acquainted with what I was putting myself through in that moment. Yet, I dismissed him based on the fact that he was a) a man and b) my father. I knew I'd made a mistake by the time he left the room.

Later, I sought him out and told him for myself that I'd found out that I was pregnant, admittedly a bit teary once again. He looked at me, full on, his attention washing over me. With no sense of judgment or value of any kind, he asked me, his voice rich and warm and slightly slowed by sleep (I'd found him after he'd taken a nap), what I wanted to do.

Each step from there followed the guideline of that question: "I" and "want" being the critical words at this particular junction. *I* decided what was best for *me* in that moment, and then the next, and then the following. At no point did my friends tell me what to do. They refrained from judgment, both negative and positive. I functioned as my own person, making decisions explicitly for me.

Eli

Just like there are socially placed limitations on how offspring-parent relationships function, there are many limits to how we are supposed to interact with the people we *do* call friends. Mainly: don't have sex with them because it's too complicated and might ruin your friendship. To some, those words will be very familiar. And if they aren't, trust me, I've heard them said plenty of times.

From my perspective, a friend is someone you tell the truth to and who tells the truth to you. Often, that kind of relationship is one of closeness because the two people actually get to know each other since they're in communication and aren't hiding parts of themselves. And because of this, I think the best people to have sex with are the ones you're friends with.

I came to adopt this viewpoint mainly through a friendship that I've built with a friend currently in my life named Eli. We first met playing soccer on the same team and eventually he moved into my intentional community. Over the time we've known each other, our relationship has looked a lot of different ways: acquaintances, boyfriend/girlfriend, partners, lovers. We've lived together, we've lived apart. But through all that, I've found that being a friend to him is the best that I can do.

This is going to start to sound pretty selfish but bear with me. I do it for me. You see, I am a friend to *him*: I tell him the truth. I do that because it feels the best to me, it's the way I feel the clearest and it's how I ensure that he knows who I am. And as it turns out, being known by another person (having someone who knows your views on life, on your sensuality, and on whatever is important to you) is liberating. That's the part from the definition of "friend" way back at the beginning of this chapter that struck me: to be a friend means to set free.

Because I feel free in my relationship with him, I'm free to tell him what I think and feel because I don't need to hide.

This conversation about friendship is a complex one, which I firmly believe could fill an entirely library if the subject were to be explored fully. My aim is to merely start a thought process which could potentially be explored further by you, dear reader. We are taught to value our spouses above our families. Our families above our friends. Our religion above all else. But I've found that exploring friendship with serious enthusiasm has expanded my life and the way I view the people in it.

But keep in mind, with friendship there is risk. The risk is twofold. The first is that when you tell them the truth, they may not like it. You may lose people: wives, acquaintances, siblings, opportunities, and experiences over this. The second is that, when you have someone as a friend, there are no guarantees. No 'til death do you part, no in sickness or in health. You can only decide to be a friend, you can't make someone else be your friend. It's the most basic form of relationship there is and also the most challenging. But there is an expansiveness, a freeness, in being a friend which has me firmly believe that the risks are well worth the reward.

Chapter 11

HOW TO TALK ABOUT THE BIRDS AND THE BEES

Earlier this year a friend of mine described the story of her ten-year-old daughter discovering her vibrator. Up until this point in their relationship my friend had been gingerly navigating the murky waters of "the talk" with her daughter. She felt that there was much she wanted to tell her, but she wasn't sure how to say it. The apparent need for the start of this conversation came to a head one morning when her daughter appeared in front of her in the living room with a bright-pink vibrator in hand, asking about this newfound item. My friend flushed bright red from head to toe while simultaneously snatching the item from her daughter's hand, and she tossed it into a nearby kitchen cupboard while calmly trying to tell her it was a back massager. Of course, her daughter then requested a back massage with the device, which my friend unfortunately had to firmly respond to with "no."

This may be a familiar story to some people, I'm sure we've all been in situations where "private" things suddenly become "public" things. I'll never forget the day I was a guest in my friend's home and my hosts' five-pound Yorkie puppy found my menstrual cup in my purse, used it as a chew toy, and then hid it under her master's bed alongside all her other favorite toys and coveted dirty socks. My friend's reaction to her daughter finding the vibrator is completely understandable, as it's natural to feel exposed in these kinds of moments. I don't think she should have done anything differently, but I do think she had an opportunity in front of her which she could have taken advantage of. Instead of reacting with shock and surprise, she could have used that moment as a way to open up a conversation about masturbation or introduce the concept of self-care through pleasure. Perhaps right after she'd tossed the dildo into the cupboard.

When people tell me they are not sure when the right time is to start these kinds of conversations, I usually feel a small degree of surprise because on one level, we're surrounded by opportunities to have these conversations in our regular, everyday lives. Those brief naked moments before hopping into the shower can be a time to mention the idea of self-care through taking care of your body. While looking in a mirror at the same time as your child, perhaps fixing your hair or straightening your tie, could be a moment to talk about approval of yourself and enjoying how you look exactly the way you are. It's these small conversations along the way that make a difference. Opportunities have a way of presenting themselves when you have the intention to talk about these things and you are paying attention to what is going on.

If you feel uncomfortable with the idea of talking to either your teen or another youth for whom you care, you're not alone. A Planned Parenthood survey found that less than 60 percent of parents felt anything more than "somewhat comfortable" at the prospect of having this kind of conversation. But it's worth persevering beyond that hesitancy as parents are still viewed, despite what one might think with the everyday availability of the Internet, as one of the most influential resources of sex education for youth. It's also important to still tackle the tough issues, as the same Planned Parenthood report[1] showed that while nearly all parents believed they were influential in whether or not their child uses birth control and condoms, just over half of parents were actually *having* those conversations.[2]

It's been shown that the key to these conversations being effective is that the conversations are ongoing. The more frequently these conversations occurred, the more open and comfortable the teen felt about discussing these topics overall. Another study concluded that repetition in discussing sexual health allowed the opportunity to "reinforce and build on what they have taught their children and provide children the opportunity to ask clarifying questions as they attempt to put their parents' sexual education into practice."[3] So please, persevere and deliberately take the time to start having conversations having to do with sexual health on an ongoing basis.

• • • • • •

The thing I get asked about most is how to bring the information that I describe in this book into a parent-child relationship. I was once interviewed for an article on having "the talk" with your teens for a well-known website and the journalist, upon my telling her about how my parents guided me through puberty and that they were still people I confided in about my life, dropped all pretense of professionalism. Our interview then switched gears completely as she began telling me about her parents and how she couldn't imagine talking to her dad about sex (and I imagine most people feel the same way). If you couldn't tell through reading the previous ten chapters of this book; I'm that person who called her dad after the first time she had intercourse just to let him know she'd done it and was happy about it. Yep, that's me. Needless to say, that article never appeared.

Whenever I tell people about what I do or about the topic of my book (which I've been writing for over three years, so this happens more than you may think), I get asked how to talk to teens about sex, but what those people are really asking for is an abridged version of what a parent should make sure to tell their kids. I usually refer to this as the Greatest Hits List version of the infamous "sex talk." This was first brought to my attention years ago when I was helping to put on an event called "Mamma Margarita Night." It was an intimate evening for the mothers of local public school students to get together, put down some cash for the school, and get wasted on sweet, tequila-heavy drinks. I was there to take coats, refill glasses, and assist in any way possible (the woman hosting the event is a close friend of mine).

Midway through the night (exactly two margaritas into the evening) one of the co-hosts of the event approached me and started some small talk about the party. Mind you, she and I had only met a mere forty-five minutes earlier, but she quickly and deftly steered the conversation toward what she really wanted to talk about: her middle-school aged daughter. Suddenly, she burst out with "I'd really like for you to spend time with my daughter." I was momentarily stunned, wondering where this could possibly be headed as her daughter was clearly beyond an age requiring babysitting. She then explained that her daughter would not talk to her about that *stuff.* This momma of two described herself as "too nerdy and too old" to be able to relate to her over sex, teenagerdom, and all those sticky topics.

It was fascinating to me that she'd try to set me up with her daughter to take care of this integral part of growing up. I think it is critical that every young person learn about their bodies, sexuality, and relationships so that they can go forth and create success in their lives. This is not a subject that I take lightly. I didn't blame this woman, as she'd hit the virtual information jackpot when she approached me about this, but I did wonder why she'd ask a total stranger to get involved. She didn't know anything about me (least of all that I was in the process of writing a sex ed book). But then I realized, that's exactly why this book needs to be written—to inform the nerdy mommas, the uninformed fourteen-year-olds, the questioners, the wonderers, the people with the equipment but no manual, the girls headed toward womanhood, the boys who want to know, and the dads who aren't quite sure what to do.

So how do you be a friend to your kid? First of all, you do not need to stop being a parent. We all know that your first job as a parent is to keep your offspring alive and keep them from doing anything too crazy, whether that's simply getting too far off track or putting themselves in mortal danger. This is not an either/or situation, it's an addition. In my view, there are three steps to add on to your relationship with your child to orient your relationship toward winning and experiencing life more pleasurably.

Step One

The first step is communicating that pleasure is good. It's part of the human experience and is something to be welcomed into your daily existence. While a seemingly simple step, it's truly an act of revolution while living in a culture that constantly communicates that pleasure is bad.

Advertising tells us we get pleasure from purchasing the products that they're slinging. We have popular phrases that are variants of the pervasive "no pain, no gain" viewpoint. But perhaps most obvious is what is acceptable and unacceptable to discuss in public settings, like at the dinner table or a cocktail party. When asked how you're doing, it's acceptable to discuss an upcoming medical procedure that is on your calendar (and thus something likely to be painful) but you'd be socially outcast if you talked about some great sex you had with your partner the previous night. Even if the latter was something much more important to you, you still shouldn't bring it up. Even talking about how good your life is, how smoothly things are running, or how happy your kids are is a less popular topic than discussing problems or painful aspects, like your bad relationship with your teenagers or how boring your job is.

Pleasure is strongly linked to sexuality and thus is relegated to private spaces or not spoken of at all. This link is purely a puritanical one and has no basis in reality. Pleasure is pleasure, it's part of the human experience. I take pleasure from the sun shining in my window, from the soft feel of my ceramic mug in my hand, and from the piercing heat of my tea penetrating the stoneware and caressing my palm. That's pleasurable. Our skin is comprised of a vast network of nerves; we are sensing organisms, but we live in a society that tells us not to feel these things or at least not acknowledge them aloud.

The change starts with you. If you're a parent, you know that children mostly learn from what they see, especially earlier on in their life. Your actions and choices create the greatest impact on how your child or even the people around you view pleasure. It's simple everyday choices that can make the greatest impact. Of course any time pleasure or sensuality comes up in conversation, you have an opportunity to reaffirm positive messages or ask questions with that intention in mind. But making regular choices to have pleasure for yourself, whether it's taking a moment in the morning to sit by the window and enjoy a cup of tea, or taking a walk outside during sunset, you can lead by example. By deliberately taking pleasure for yourself and having that be a positive experience, you demonstrate to others that pleasure is good and something to be deliberately sought out.

• • • • • •

"Can you do this?" she asked, excitedly, as she brought her foot next to her curl-covered head with her skinny leg completely outstretched, other foot firmly planted on the wet pool deck. Pondering her position from the pool, I frowned and declined. I've never been able to touch my own toes in a forward bend; I certainly could not "do that." Laying back in the water, I quickly completed a backwards somersault and retorted, "Can you do that?" Ignoring me, she spun several times sideways in the water, a blur of shiny-purple swimsuit and limbs, and said, "I can do that, can you?" once she emerged. Nodding with confidence, I followed suit and spun on my side, mirroring her as best I could. This session of "Can You Do This?" went on for another twenty minutes at least, as we each demonstrated feats of our own athletic abilities; cartwheels, more leg stretches, underwater bridge-pose. It didn't matter to either of us that we were two decades and at least eighty pounds apart. The light competition and intensive mimicry was fun and completely absorbing. A dash of showing off mixed with raw athleticism and performance, the time flew by. Before that afternoon in the pool, we'd barely spent longer than ten seconds looking at one another, let alone talking. At the same baby shower, but for totally different reasons; she the daughter of the aunt-to-be and me the partner of the uncle-to-be, we didn't have a lot of common ground. But we certainly found it in the pool.

A month later, as I was riding my bike through the Mission District, that hot afternoon in the pool came to mind and I suddenly realized that moment was a perfect example of how humans learn. Simply put: we watch each other do stuff. As an awkward teen, I figured out how to dress by watching the other students in my classes at community college. When I first started playing soccer, I figured out how to do it by watching the good players do their thing and mimicking what I could. We are constantly teaching other people by how we behave and the choices we make, just as we are constantly gathering information and learning from the people in our environment.

Step Two

The second component is what I call "vocabulary." Peggy Orenstein argues in her enlightening book *Girls & Sex* that we must give children, particularly girls, vocabulary for their genitals. We tend to not name things that we are uncomfortable or unaccustomed to talking about, and this shows up no more prominently than in relation to the genitalia of females.[4] With boys, this is less of an issue. They've got peters, puds, dicks, cocks, johnsons, tools, and willies; plenty of cute names to safely refer to the penis. The term "penis" itself is even pretty safe to say aloud in polite society. It's medicalized just enough that one can say it without fear of consequence. However, the equivalent term for girls, "vulva," is virtually unknown. We tend to use the term "vagina" even though that word actually describes the interior portion of the female reproductive system, the portion in between the cervix and introitus. There are a few other terms used to refer to the female genitalia, but they tend to be viewed as more crass and are considered unacceptable terms. Alternatively, we have a good number of objects that we use to describe or refer to a person's vulva, like purse, clam, or pocket, which are terribly oblique, refer to something "closed," and reek of objectification.

Research has shown that the difference between how girls' and boys' bodies are represented goes further than our common speech and can be found reflected in the dictionaries that are provided to youth for their education. John Willinsky explored this topic and demonstrated how different dictionaries completely omitted the clitoris in their definitions, and he also described other attempts in dictionaries to erase female sexuality completely from the very works which should be starting places for education and illumination.[5]

Orenstein points out that by not naming girls' genitals, or even worse, only referring to them as "private parts," we rob them of a means to communicate and we make their genitals unmentionable. Why do we give them names for their chin, their elbow, and their pinky toenail, but not a part that is so central to their everyday experience? Not just in terms of pleasure, but in basic everyday bodily functions. After all, one of the first things we are ever trained to do is pee in a potty as opposed to just going in our diaper.

So, a major step is to give all the body parts words and make those words acceptable and safe to use. Children learn by mimicking, so however you feel about those words will be emulated by them. Your confidence and rightness in speaking about your and their body will have a tangible effect.

Further than simply naming body parts is opening up the lines of communication. By fostering a conversation around the body, you can introduce an ongoing topic of conversation between you and your child. I think Peggy Orenstein's point is representative of a larger aim of not only giving girls and boys terms to use for their own bodies, but opening up a larger highway of information where questions are met with acceptance and answers, sensitive or challenging topics are broached and openly discussed, and a sense of openness and rapport is established.

Since my mom talked to me freely about her body as well as mine, I felt comfortable going to her when I had questions or concerns. In an earlier chapter, I told a story about my concerns over not being able to find my clitoris, which is an amusing story to look back on, but at the same time I wonder what could have happened if I hadn't been able to talk—or felt uncomfortable talking to—my mom? How would I have been able to access that information? I don't have an answer for those questions, but I know I am immensely grateful that I grew up in a place where those lines of communication were open and available to me.

Step Three

The third component is approval. This is a tricky one for a lot of people. I view approving of others in a similar way to what we discussed in the earlier chapter on body image. Approving of what you see in the mirror, or when you look down at your body, is a choice. Some days it may be easier to like what you see than others, but each moment is an opportunity to make a new decision.

Here are some keys to approving: you don't have to like something to approve of it and, secondly, you can approve of anything. Yes, even that horrible thing you just thought of. It's possible. I'm not saying that I do it all of the time and in every single circumstance, but it is a tool that I use every day.

There is another viewpoint that closely relates to the subject of approval that could also be a useful tool. In driver's education we all learned that it's best to turn in the same direction that you are already turning if you begin to lose control of the car while driving in icy conditions or skidding for another reason. It seems counter-intuitive, but it's the most effective way to regain control of the car. Approving of the people around you and being in agreement with their actions are two key concepts in building friendlier relationships with the people in your life.

My Dad told me when I was a kid that his definition of love is "intense approval." This affected me in two ways. The first is that it simplified the concept of love for me. Once I took on this definition as my own, love no longer felt like this giant, mysterious entity that I'd heard mythologized in pop songs and in books. It became something that I could choose to do at will and that others could choose for themselves. It also changed my concept of approval. I began seeing that when I approved of another person or thing, it would begin to feel like that strong, deep emotion I associated with loving. From there, approval began to look like a tool, a building block. It's one step in the direction of good and if you keep approving of someone for long enough or with enough intensity, you may just end up loving that person.

Approving doesn't mean you tell your kid that everything they do is right. Letting them do everything they think of and approving of them are not synonymous concepts. In fact, one of the best examples of a time in my life when my dad approved of me was during a time when I felt like I was at my worst.

He called me at night, which was the first sign that things were off. This was the early 2000s and while I had a cell phone, I rarely used it to make calls because I was limited to around 300 minutes a month (remember those days?). We talked frequently, but it was often through a message app or through webcam chats with my sister at my side, and it was rarely just the two of us on a phone call.

My sister and I had moved to our family home in San Francisco to attend college. Respectively, we were only seventeen and sixteen, but since we'd already finished up the homeschool equivalent of high school, it felt like the next natural step to continue our formal education. But as it turns out, I still had a lot of growing up to do.

Since I was sixteen, I figured that I was basically an adult and had it all figured out for myself. I look back on those years and usually cringe silently to myself. I acted overly self-confident with absolutely no true confidence and by feeling like I had everything figured out, I demonstrated with absolute skill that I was yet a baby in the grand scope of life. I was on a soccer team and fell in with those women as if they were my idols I should replicate my own life after, when they barely had their own lives figured out. Every boy that I batted my eyelashes at felt like an opportunity to pursue. I began to lose myself in that maze of new experiences, people, and choices. This showed up the most in my relationships with the people I was closest with. Conversations with my mom became shorter and shorter as I turned away from her and looked toward these new people. I became difficult and demanding with the people I lived beside, putting unreasonable expectations on them one minute and ignoring them the next. I started to change, physically and personality-wise. My grades started slipping; I flunked a beginning French exam simply because I thought I didn't need to study for it.

Hearing my dad's voice on the other end of the line, I knew something was up. He's not a showy speaker and his conversations are devoid of filler words, no um's or uh's; he's not one to let you off the hook with extraneous verbiage. He quickly got to the point and told me that this just wasn't working out and that he wanted me to come home for the next semester. At those words, it felt like my whole world caved in. I sat down on the two carpet-covered steps near my feet. Enclosed in the darkened room, I looked down at the ground to consider what he'd said. It left no room for argument and without doubt shattered my illusions of independence and adulthood. I knew I'd do what he said. I asked if I could finish the semester out, since we were right before our mid-semester break for Thanksgiving. He replied in the affirmative and I disconnected the call.

The worst part was the embarrassment. I'd carefully crafted my image as an adult, as someone forging her own path in this wild city of San Francisco. I was a significant player on the school soccer team, I had a full-time student workload, and I was beginning to take over the food program and nonprofit organization that my intentional community ran. I had all the makings of being a fully-grown woman, but suddenly I was being told what to do by my dad all over again.

I was not happy with him about this for quite a while, years really. I went home for that semester, which then turned into a year. While I went through the motions of being a contributing part of the household, I had this thorn in my side about him telling me what to do. After a couple of months of that rather depressive behavior, my dad came into my room one morning and asked me what I was going to do that day. A visit from my dad in my room was pretty rare and was enough to make me sit up straight and scramble for a plan. I didn't have one. The project I came up with related to fixing one of the many nuances of my own bedroom. He said he'd had enough of the way I'd been choosing to act and told me I had to find something to do, anything, that was for the group. Again, I felt embarrassed at my dad barging into my life and telling me what to do but, this time, I also began to realize how much attention I had on myself and how little I had for other people.

From there, I began to look outward, which for me meant physically going outside and becoming engaged. I rediscovered the multitude of projects, chores, and daily activities that kept our twenty-plus-acre piece of property running smoothly. I picked up my previous charge as chicken lady, which meant evening visits to the poultry yard to feed and care for our flock of fifty hens and handful of roosters, guinea fowl, and turkeys. Tromping down the rolling hill that led to our aptly named "lower garden" and chicken yard clad in oversized sky-blue Dickies coveralls and bulky muck boots, I started to become attuned to and build awareness of the goings-on that surrounded me: a dozen adults living together while simultaneously raising our own food, raising two toddlers, and facilitating regular retreats and courses based on the information we lived by.

Meetings, frequent one-on-one conversations, and deliberate attention on each other is what kept us in such efficient harmony and, gradually, I became a part of this once more. Over the next few years as I steadily grew into a woman, I began to talk more about my daily experience: what I was feeling, who I was thinking about, what I noticed, and what I wanted. I realized that I had a network of people in front of me who only wanted me to succeed. The people I had taken for my oppressors, the ones calling me up on any given evening and telling me what to do, I began to realize were my greatest assets: they were my friends.

I would not have gotten to this point if it were not for approval, or more specifically, my family's deliberate choice to approve of me. There were times when I was a raving bitch, storming through the house, tossing expletives and slamming doors, but along the way I still had people who viewed me as a totally adequate human being. That's what allowed me to talk when I was ready: they created a safe space for me to say what I needed to say without fear of consequence or repercussion.

• • • • • •

The three components that I have just described—practicing pleasure, opening up vocabulary, and being approving—are the key aspects for creating positive, long-lasting relationships with the people that are important to you. While I've discussed these viewpoints from the perspective of a parent raising a child, these are actually tools that work for any relationship that's important to you. From my perspective, these conversations are a two-way street for the parents and the children, or youth with their friends, or parents/guardians with one another (whatever combination applies to you, dear reader) to have the kinds of communications and quality of relationships that they each want to have.

Some people feel that there are certain topics that will always be off limits, no matter what. But I've found that even some of the most personal, emotionally charged aspects of our lives, like birth and death, can be communicated about clearly and effectively, for the betterment of everyone around.

· · · · · ·

When I was five years old, I walked into the bathroom while Julia, one of the women who lived in the house and with whom I was very close, was sitting on the toilet. This was pretty common practice. I frequently visited my friends while they relieved themselves; I even recall sitting on my mom's lap a time or two while she took a poop, only scooting off of her when she was finished and ready to wipe. Yes, as a kid I had absolutely *no* boundaries when it came to people's privacy or personal preferences. That morning, I could sense that things were different. Julia's face was ashen when she looked up at me from her perch on the cool, white commode. I asked her what was happening and when she didn't respond immediately, I left to return a few minutes later, still curious. This time I saw it. A small blob of red tissue roughly the size of a lime sitting in the toilet bowl. She told me that it was going to be a baby, but it'd come out of her instead. I was puzzled by this, of course, but from the level tone she was using I concluded that while she was certainly sad, she was okay.

That was the first time I learned about miscarriage. When the topic has come up since then, I often flashback to that memory: Julia's matter-of-fact description of what had happened, the slight melancholy that infused the room and matched the yellowish pallor that the morning light colored our bathroom. It wasn't until many years later that I realized the profoundness of that moment, to which there are many parts. The first being that she actually told me what had happened. Miscarriage, the loss of a pregnancy, is a highly taboo topic in our culture which consequently means very few are willing to discuss the experience.

The second component of what made that moment with Julia unique is that she told me what was happening in a calm, level fashion without emotion added in a situation which was certainly not a positive one for her. Miscarriage is often a negative experience for people and can bring feelings of sadness or even guilt at the loss. Had Julia cried or been angry when she told me, that would have changed my perception of miscarriage itself. Or further, had she tried to play it off like she was actually happy when she wasn't, that too would have altered how I perceived the experience. Instead, she told me the truth and I concluded that it was a natural part of her experience and thus, a natural part of life.

• • • • • •

Talking about "the birds and the bees" is not easy for everyone, in fact, it comes to very few naturally. Even though I was raised by sex educators who did everything they could to instill in me the concept that my body is good, that pleasure is a natural part of life, and that none of these topics are anything to be ashamed about, I have still had my own challenges. It wasn't until I reached my mid-twenties that I could stand to say the word "masturbation" directly and with confidence, instead of using slang or coded language. The first time I talked to my friends about the pleasurable experiences I had, there were things I felt perfectly open to talking about, and then there were things that felt more uncomfortable and challenging. I had my own reaching to do. If you find talking about sensuality or sexuality difficult: you're not alone. My goal is to encourage you to press forward, beyond the discomfort, to create an open dialogue between you and your confidant.

CONCLUSION

Navigating the path from adolescence into adulthood is not necessarily easy. It seems a common experience is one of being carefully raised and nurtured by parents and guardians at the start of life and through childhood, but as we draw nearer to our teens and the threshold of adulthood, which is somewhat arbitrarily designated to be eighteen in the United States, that guidance begins to shift. Instead of intently guiding this aspect of growth and transition, a more "hands-off" approach is sometimes adopted and sex ed is left to the school system or is something you are just supposed to know how to do innately when the time comes. Sometimes in the throes of puberty, relationships between guardians and teens can become so strained and challenging that one or the other deems it necessary to sever the relationship. Or, the parting of ways comes in the less dramatic yet equally separating experience of leaving the family home to begin college or to enter the workforce. Although this form of separation is socially acceptable, it's still a severing of ties. I've heard many parents comment on their feelings of "empty nest" or refer to how their child is "on their own now." From my perspective, turning eighteen or moving away are not the kinds of events that warrant a complete divide between the guiding force of parents and their offspring. I am not sure this severance need occur in the way I typically see it transpire.

I see becoming an adult as more of a time of transition, a period of blossoming.

You are a role model, whether you've admitted that to yourself or not. Each of us affects the people around us, whether we live with them or sit beside them at our desks. The choices that you make have an effect on others. If you are in the role of a parent, guardian, and caregiver, you can model *pleasure* and *happiness* for the people that you have the greatest impact on (your kids), regardless of their age. By "modeling pleasure" I mean that you can value it in your own life and impact others through your own value system. *Pleasure* is one of those words that we sometimes associate with sexuality; "self-pleasure," after all is merely the nicer-sounding version of the rather clinical term "masturbation," for example. But that's not the only sense that I mean of the word. It's far greater than that.

Pleasure in the sense that has been used in this book is more about taking in what's around you through your senses and experiencing enjoyment. That can be in a sensual or sexual setting, but further than that it can be in your day-to-day life. Taking a moment to savor what you're eating, feeling the texture of your clothes against your body, or appreciating the play of sunlight against a building. These are seemingly tiny moments in our lives that, when noticed, can lead to a greater experience of happiness and enjoyment. And in turn, this affects the people around us.

Another critical aspect of leading a pleasurable life (as that *has* been the secret objective of this book all along), is clear communication. In truth, to say "clear" alongside "communication" is a redundancy, since a communication has only truly occurred if it's been clearly made, but I add that word on to make a distinction between being deliberate and operating by default. Many people communicate as if they are not entirely in control of what is said and the ultimate outcome of their actions. But as outlined in the previous chapter, through approaching your communications with intention, you can have the kinds of conversations and, consequently, the kinds of relationships you want to surround yourself with.

The bedroom is one of those places where it's easy to believe that words have no place, or at least that the rules of communication are different. There is an abundance of social rules and stigma around talking during sensual activities. But in my view, speaking in an intimate setting doesn't have to be different than the communications we have in other important settings. Using the tools outlined earlier, like asking winning questions and using the tool of safe porting, will make all of your communications better. You'll get what you want out of the experiences you create and you will have fun doing it.

Clear communication is a key aspect to building positive relationships, perhaps never more so than with our friends and family. The friendships we hold, that is, those relationships in which we tell the truth, are immensely valuable since that is a place where we can be most wholly ourselves. You can be friends with anyone you want, whether or not you already have a relationship with them. Some of my closest friends are actually people that play other roles in my life, like "mother" or "sister," but because I have chosen to treat them like friends, our relationships have grown to mean more to me and add more into my life.

Knowing how to have these kinds of conversations can be challenging. There is no one-size-fits-all for sex education. Nor are there guidelines to simply look up a topic and know exactly what to say and how to say it. I am confident though that anyone who is willing to talk about human sexuality and use the tools described, whether it is about their own experience or as a way to guide someone, will find the words. All I aim to do is provide a path on which to navigate through the vast woods we call "adulthood."

RESOURCES FOR CONTINUED EDUCATION

Welcome to the Resources portion of this book. My focus thus far has been on describing the difference between sensuality and sexuality in a practical sense: how to make choices for your pleasure and how to lead a life that is sex-positive, communicative, and is centered on friendship. The rest of this chapter goes over some of the fundamentals of adulting and taking care of your body: how to use a health clinic, birth control options, additional resources for sex education, an overview of STIs (sexually transmitted infections), and an explanation of a great tool called "safe-porting."

Using a Clinic

There are several options available for health and medical assistance. If you are insured through your parents, you can visit a doctor through their medical services. Even if you are using their insurance, you can request that your services are kept private. If it is their policy to inform parents of your visit, you can seek out services at a public health clinic. Planned Parenthood is one of many types of clinics available. Using an online resource like TeenSource.com can help you find a clinic in your area. If you go to public school, you can also utilize your school's health services. Generally speaking, doctors have a policy of confidentiality with their patient, which means that any services or tests you have done will be kept between you and the clinic itself. In order to encourage you to seek the care you need, there are laws in place to make sure you have access to confidential medical services which include (but are not limited to): birth control (including emergency contraception, like Plan B), STI testing and treatment for STIs (ages twelve and over), pregnancy tests and prenatal care, abortion procedures, and mental health services. You can always call ahead to ask about a clinic's confidentiality practice and check to see if they provide the services you require.

It's important to begin seeing a doctor once you reach your early teens (thirteen to fifteen) in order to stay healthy and ensure you're protected from STIs and other health issues. Both men and women can visit a doctor regularly for checkups. A typical visit to a gynecologist (a doctor that specializes in women's reproductive health) may include a series of exams, specifically a pelvic exam and breast exam. It could also include: testing for STIs (usually through a small blood draw and a urine test), a pap smear, and any vaccines you may need. A pelvic exam is when a doctor looks at your genitals and reproductive organs, like your vulva, vagina, uterus, ovaries, and fallopian tubes. A pap smear usually occurs after you've turned twenty-one, but sometimes can happen earlier. This exam is where your cervix is swabbed for cells which are tested for abnormalities. Men can visit a general doctor for regular checkups, which could include an overall physical exam as well as testicular and breast exam, in addition to an STI screening. If the general doctor finds something of concern, they may make a recommendation to see a urologist (a doctor who specializes in male reproductive health). If you are experiencing any ongoing pain or notice unusual changes in your genital areas (i.e., changes in odor or discoloration), you should talk to your doctor immediately.

I visited a doctor specifically for my own sexual health when I was in my early teens to have certain questions answered about symptoms I'd noticed in my genital region. I had never had sexual contact at that point, but it was important for me to seek out assistance with the conditions that I'd observed. The care I received was professional and the doctor readily answered my questions.

Years later, when I first began having intercourse, I decided to go to Planned Parenthood for my first exam and to have bloodwork done for STI testing, even though I'd had protected sex. I felt that it was important to begin getting tested because I intended to be sexually active and wanted to maintain my health. As I got older, and began visiting a health clinic more regularly, I became more familiar and relaxed in the setting and came to appreciate what a great resource it was. Most of my appointments have been free or low-cost and even though I have not had a regular nurse or doctor (one that I have seen each time I visited), I have always found the people who treated me to be considerate and forthcoming with information whenever I asked, and even when I didn't.

I felt pretty surprised by my first pap smear. It seemed very strange to me that a doctor would even be looking at my genitals directly; at the time I barely did that myself. It's perfectly fine to be nervous, but know that you can ask any questions you have and if you feel unsafe, you can stop the exam.

Health Clinics

You can access sexual health experts through several different means: your school, your regular doctor, or through a number of public clinics. There are many online resources to help you find a nearby clinic that provides the services you require. Some of these sites are listed here:

Bedsider (Birth Control only, in the United States):
    https://www.bedsider.org/where_to_get_it
Planned Parenthood (within the United States):
    https://www.plannedparenthood.org/health-center
Stay Teen (within the United States):
    http://stayteen.org/health-centers/search
Health Link BC (Canada):
    https://www.healthlinkbc.ca/services-and-resources/find-services

Other Great Resources for Sexual Education

The research and development around sexuality, sensuality, and how to live a pleasurable, healthy life is a big field. In my research, I have found several people that are true standouts. Googling anything about sex or health is a pretty risky business as much of what is available online is negative and pain-oriented. I think much of what propels people to get online and write is negative charge and emotions. It can be useful to directly seek out people and resources that are value-neutral and are aimed towards winning and pleasure.

Heather Corinna, author of *S.E.X.: The All-You-Need-to-Know Sexuality Guide to Get You through Your Teens and Twenties* and founder of Scarleteen (www.scarleteen.com)

Corinna is one of the best resources for straightforward, sex-positive information about sex, relationships, and reproductive health. She pushes an inclusive, balanced agenda when it comes to sex ed and I highly recommend both the online resource and the book.

Planned Parenthood (PP)

Most people have probably heard of PP by now, but in case you haven't, or in case you don't know what they're about, check out their website: www .plannedparenthood.com/. PP provides many useful services in the fields of family planning, sexual health, and women's reproductive health. You can go online to request assistance or make an appointment (you can also call), or you can explore their online resources covering a range of topics, including STIs, gender and sexual identity, sex, and wellness.

The Welcomed Consensus

Formed in 1992, The Welcomed Consensus is comprised of eight individuals who teach courses on the topics of communication, sensuality, and relationships. They offer courses, instructional videos, as well as online content for adult education.

Sex, Etc. (www.sexetc.org)

This is a user-friendly website created by and for teenagers with information on topics ranging from birth control, anatomy, relationships, sex myths, gender and LGBTQ awareness and support, how to start a conversation with a parent or adult about sexual health, and more. Additionally, they provide other resources about how to find an STI testing center near you, a blog about current events related to sexual health, forums to openly ask the questions you have about sexual health and relationships, and fun educational games to test your knowledge about safer sex.

Amaze (www.amaze.org)

This website features inclusive animated videos on a wide range of topics including puberty, male and female anatomy, sexual orientation, personal safety, pregnancy and reproduction, STIs, and healthy relationships. Similarly, they provide a list of resources and videos for educators and parents, including starting points for conversations about masturbation, puberty, and relationships, and scripts for parents to follow to have a series of conversations about sexual health.

The Body Is Not an Apology:
Radical Self-Love for Everybody and Every Body
(https://thebodyisnotanapology.com)

This site has short videos, articles, and resources on topics including weight, gender, race, mental health, aging, and intersections of these variations. As well as being a good resource to learn more about these topics, there is a community platform to connect with other people who are also body positive. They have a particular focus on social media and ways to shift a culture of shaming to "radical self love" for teens and adults alike.

Family Planning and Contraception

Planned Parenthood, as I described previously, is an excellent resource for questions regarding pregnancy, whether wanted or unwanted. There are several hotlines available for immediate information, as well:

Emergency Contraception Information: 1-888-NOT-2-LATE

National Abortion Federation Hotline: 1-800-772-9100

Planned Parenthood: 1-800-230-PLAN

Pregnancy Helpline: 1-800-848-5683

Scarleteen Crisis Text Line: 1-206-866-2279

I highly recommend talking to someone close to you about the choices you are making in regard to your body; whether that's about your sexual health, experiences you are considering having, or any questions you may have. This could be a range of people, depending on your situation: parents, teachers, guardians, or a person that you feel willing to open up to.

And, keep in mind that in California and in many US states, you have the right to privacy with your healthcare, regardless of your age. Doctors are required by law to ask for your permission before releasing any of your personal information. Even if you use your parents' healthcare or are on someone else's insurance, you can still request that your information is kept private. This is in place to remove the stigma around our sexual health and to encourage everyone to use the health services that are available. The only exception is if your health care provider believes that you are putting yourself or another person in danger, or if you are having sex with a person and there is a considerable age difference. To learn more about your reproductive health rights, check out http://teenhealthlaw.org/resources-links/.

Birth Control

There are many safe, reliable forms of birth control available for a range of costs. The online resource Bedsider.com is by far the best website I've found for information about birth control methods. I highly recommend exploring their site to help you find the right method for you. I also recommend talking to your healthcare provider to help in your decision-making process.

Some methods require more forethought than others (like making an appointment to have an Intra-Uterine Device [IUD] inserted) while others require daily or weekly maintenance (like the pill). Inner and outer condoms are the only method that prevent pregnancy as well as provide STI protection. Besides abstinence, no other form of birth control provides a physical barrier between bodily fluids, so I recommend using both a form of birth control (whether that's an IUD, the pill, or any other form of contraception) in addition to using latex barriers.

Next you will find a short summary of some of the most effective and recommended forms of birth control. Please visit the aforementioned website or a site like Planned Parenthood and talk to your healthcare provider for a more comprehensive list.

• • • • • •

IUD (Intra-Uterine Device): This is basically a tiny (less than one inch long) plastic "T" that is inserted into the uterus. IUDs come in both hormonal and nonhormonal varieties. The nonhormonal type, the Paraguard (which is the only type of nonhormonal IUD available in the United States), contains a small amount of copper which creates a sufficiently inhospitable environment for an embryo to implant on the uterine lining, which prevents pregnancy. There are four main types of hormonal IUD available in the US (namely Mirena, Skyla, Liletta, and Kyleena) all of which work by releasing a small amount of the hormone progestin into the body which thickens the cervical mucus and prevents sperm from reaching the egg. This device must be inserted and removed by a healthcare provider. Once it is inserted, the wearer is immediately safe from pregnancy, and once the IUD is removed, the person is able to get pregnant very soon, if not immediately. IUDs are long-lasting: depending on the brand and type you select you can be protected from three to twelve years.[1]

• • • • • •

Implant: With this method, a tiny rod is inserted into the arm. It stays below the surface of the skin and is essentially invisible. The device releases a hormone that keeps your ovaries from releasing eggs and thickens your cervical mucus—which prevents sperm from getting to the egg in the first place. Like the IUD, this method is virtually undetectable and keeps your choice private. It is also long-lasting; once implanted, the device will be effective for up to four years.[2]

• • • • • •

The Shot, the Patch, the Ring, and the Pill: All four of these methods are a form of hormonal birth control and work by varying the levels of the hormones estrogen and progesterone, stopping the release of eggs and thickening the cervical mucus, which prevents sperm from reaching the egg. The 'Shot' is given every three months, while the patch has hormones emebedded in an adhesive sticker that is applied to the body (you can place the patch on your buttocks, upper outer arm, lower abdomen or upper body), usually once a week. The ring consists of plastic that is embedded with hormones, which is placed inside the vagina to sit around the cervix, and is replaced monthly. The pill is an oral method of hormonal birth control, meaning you take a pill once a day at the same time. It is important to take the pill regularly, as skipping a daily dose of hormones may not be effective at preventing an egg from being released, and can lead to pregnancy if no other form of contraception is being used. None of these methods are available over the counter, but all are available through a health provider.[3]

· · · · · ·

Condoms: With proper use, they are 98 percent effective against pregnancy and are the most effective prevention against most types of STIs.[4] They are an excellent additional safety net if one is already using another form of pregnancy prevention. Condoms come in a variety of materials (both latex and nonlatex are common), flavors, and textures, and some even have spermicide (a cream, gel, or foam that contains chemicals which kill sperm) added for extra protection.[5]

STI (Sexually Transmitted Infections) Information

Sex is great and all, but it's a dangerous world out there and we must take steps to protect ourselves and be deliberate, especially when it comes to partnered sex. This is a partial list of known STIs (sexually transmitted infections) for your education and reference. It is by no means a comprehensive list or meant to replace a visit to an actual doctor. If you know that you have had exposure to an STI or think that you may be at risk, please seek immediate medical assistance.

Being proactive with your health and wellness is essential. All of the below information on STIs is from the text *Human Sexuality in a World of Diversity*, besides where otherwise noted.[6]

STIs include a range of health issues that are passed from person to person via sexual contact and/or swapping of bodily fluids. The main bodily fluids that transmit STIs are cervical mucus, semen, and blood. Some STIs can be transmitted through breast milk and saliva, as well. Some STIs are treatable, while others are not.[7]

It's important to listen to your body and note any changes you may experience. Unusual discharge (in color or smell) from your vagina or penis or irritation can be a sign that you should seek medical help. It's always better to call a medical center than let symptoms go untreated.

Viruses

Viruses are protein-coated particles of DNA incapable of reproducing on their own. In order for a virus to reproduce, or replicate, it must enter a living cell and hijack the cell's replication machinery to make more copies of the viral DNA. As more copies of the viral DNA are made and released into the body, other cells are infected. Viral STIs are treatable, but not curable, meaning it is possible to manage symptoms, but once the virus is in your body, it stays there. Some viral STIs are HIV (the virus that causes AIDS), HPV, hepatitis, and herpes.[8]

HIV/AIDS

HIV (Human Immunodeficiency Virus) is the virus that causes AIDS. This virus attacks the body's immune system, which normally defends the body from harmful organisms. A person who has a certain concentration of HIV in their body can develop AIDS (Acquired Immunodeficiency Syndrome) which affects a person's ability to fend off harmful bacteria, fungi, and other viruses a healthy immune system normally would.[9]

HIV is transmitted through bodily fluids including blood, semen, vaginal fluids, and breast milk. Transmission can occur during unprotected vaginal, anal, and oral sex, as well any means of blood transfer like sharing needles (for medical use like steroid, hormone, or insulin shots, or recreational purposes like intravenous drug use, body piercing, or tattooing) with an infected person, or an open wound or cut, including micro-abrasions in mucus membranes in or around the genitals. It is possible to transmit HIV through genital/hand contact if a person has a hangnail or micro-abrasions on their hands or fingers. However, HIV cannot be transmitted through day-to-day contact like hugging, shaking hands, using the toilet, or sitting on a couch.[10]

As previously mentioned, once a person is infected with HIV there is no cure. However, there is medication that can manage symptoms and decrease the chance of transmitting the virus to another person. Prevention is far more affordable than treatments to manage HIV/AIDS.

HPV

Human Papillomavirus, or HPV, is the most common STI.[11] There are over forty types of HPV.[12] The two main symptoms of a HPV infection are genital warts and cervical cancer. Genital warts are itchy bumps that can be different sizes, shapes, and colors depending on where they occur. In women, genital warts can appear on the vulva, on the vaginal wall, and in the cervix. For men, genital warts can be on the penis, foreskin, scrotum, or in the urethra. There are also other areas where HPV-caused genital warts can occur, including the mouth, on the lips, eyelids, nipples, anus, or in the rectum.[13] Additionally, HPV was present in 94 percent of cervical cancer tumors tested.[14] However, it is common for no symptoms to occur and a person can spread the infection without knowing it.[15]

Transmission of HPV can occur through skin-to-skin contact during vaginal, anal, or oral sex. Other forms of contact, such as touching an infected towel or clothing can also transmit the virus. However, there is currently a vaccine available called Gardasil which can make most women and men immune to HPV.[16] Similarly, people with healthy immune systems can clear most HPV infections naturally. The most common method for detection of HPV in women is through a pap smear. There are currently no HPV tests for men, however, since genital warts are a sign of HPV a visual screening by a doctor can indicate the presence of HPV in a male.

Treating genital warts is most commonly done with cryotherapy, or freezing off the wart with liquid nitrogen. There are also other chemical treatments available for managing genital warts.[17]

Hepatitis

There are four main types of hepatitis: A, B, C, and D. Hepatitis affects the liver, which becomes inflamed when infected. A person with a hepatitis infection often does not have any symptoms. However, some symptoms can include a loss of appetite, abdominal discomfort, whitish bowel movements, and brownish urine.[18]

Hepatitis can be transmitted in a variety of ways. Hepatitis A is transmitted through infected fecal matter contaminating food or water, as well as oral-anal sex. Hepatitis B can be sexually transmitted through anal, vaginal, or oral sex with an infected partner, as well as contact with contaminated blood, saliva, nasal mucus, or semen. It is possible to transmit hepatitis B through sharing razors, toothbrushes, or other personal articles with an infected person. Similarly, hepatitis C and D are sexually transmitted or passed on through contact with contaminated blood. Hepatitis D only occurs in the presence of hepatitis B.[19]

There is no cure for hepatitis. However, there is a vaccine called Dynavax for hepatitis B. There is also a vaccine for hepatitis A. There is no vaccine for hepatitis C.[20]

Herpes

Genital herpes is caused by the herpes simplex 2 virus, or HSV-2, while oral herpes is caused by the herpes simplex 1 virus, or HSV-1. Oral herpes causes cold sores or fever blisters on the mouth and lips and can be transferred to the genitals during oral sex. Genital herpes is characterized by blisters and shallow sores on the genitals. Once a person is infected with the herpes virus, it remains dormant in their body in the nerve cells in the base of the spine. Stress can lower the immune system's functions, triggering an outbreak of sores.[21]

Both types of herpes viruses can be transmitted through direct and indirect contact. Oral herpes can be transmitted through kissing (direct) or sharing a cup (indirect) with an infected person. Genital herpes can also be directly transmitted through intercourse, oral sex, or anal sex, and indirectly through sharing a towel with an infected person. The most contagious time is during an outbreak when sores on the mouth or genitals are visible. However, it is still possible to transmit the virus between outbreaks. Herpes can be spread from one part of the body to an uninfected part of the body by touching the sore and then touching another part of the body, for instance the eyes, causing ocular herpes.[22]

Though there is no cure for herpes, there are treatments and vaccines available.

Bacterial Infections

Bacteria are single-celled microorganisms that are prevalent in the environment, as well as in and on our bodies. Many types of bacteria are beneficial and essential for maintaining a healthy body, particularly in our digestive systems. However, there are some types of bacteria that are harmful and cause diseases such as pneumonia, tuberculosis, and STIs including gonorrhea, syphilis, and chlamydia.[23] Most bacterial infections are treatable with antibiotics. However, there are strains of bacteria that have become resistant to antibiotic treatments, which is why it is important to only take antibiotics when they are prescribed by a doctor.

Gonorrhea

Gonorrhea, also known as "the clap," is caused by a gonococcus bacterium. Like many bacteria, gonococcal bacteria grow in moist, warm environments like the mucous membranes of the urinary tract in both men and women, as well as on the cervix in women. Symptoms of gonorrhea in men include a yellowish discharge from the penis and painful urination. For women, the symptoms are similar and include increased vaginal discharge, painful urination, or irregular menstruation. Symptoms may not appear until five days after infection.[24]

Gonorrhea is transmitted through the exchange of bodily fluids during unprotected vaginal, anal, or oral sex. It is possible to transmit the bacteria that causes gonorrhea to a person's throat during oral sex, resulting in pharyngeal gonorrhea. Gonorrhea is more likely to be spread through penile discharge than vaginal discharge, and is highly contagious.[25]

Once gonorrhea is diagnosed through a clinical inspection of the genitals and a culture of genital discharge, it can be treated with a standard course of antibiotics.

Syphilis

Syphilis is caused by a spiral-shaped bacterium called *Treponema pallidum*. Syphilis progresses through several stages of infection that have different symptoms. In the first stage, two to four weeks after infection, a painless chancre or sore develops. Chancres form on infected mucous membranes or skin abrasions. The second stage of syphilis can occur up to a few months after the initial infection. This secondary stage is characterized by a skin rash of reddish, painless, raised bumps that burst and release a discharge. Other symptoms of this stage include sores on the mouth, a sore throat, painful swelling of the joints, headaches, and fever. Once these symptoms disappear, syphilis enters the latent stage where it can lay dormant for up to forty years. After a period of being dormant, syphilis will enter the third, or tertiary, stage, which is characterized by an ulcer on the digestive organs, on the skin, muscle tissue, lungs, liver, or other organs.[26]

Syphilis is most commonly transmitted through vaginal or anal intercourse, or oral sex with the genitals and/or the anus of an infected person. Transmission of the bacteria can also happen when a person's mucous membranes or skin abrasions come in contact with the open sores of an infected person.[27]

Diagnosis of syphilis usually occurs in the first stage with a clinical examination of the fluid from a sore. A blood test is effective once the infection has entered the secondary stage. Syphilis is treated with antibiotics, usually penicillin, though there are other options for those who are allergic to penicillin.[28]

Chlamydia

Chlamydia is another common bacterial STI caused by a parasitic bacterium that can only survive within cells. The bacterium *Chlamydia trachomatis* can cause a number of infections in both men and women, mostly in internal structures like the urethra, the epididymis in men, and the cervix in women. In men, symptoms include a thin, whitish discharge from the penis, and sometimes burning or painful urination. The scrotum and testes may also feel sore or heavy. In women, they may also feel a burning sensation during urination or a mild vaginal discharge, as well as an irregular menstrual cycle. In untreated women, the infection can spread into the reproductive system and cause sterility.[29]

The most common ways chlamydia is transmitted is through vaginal or anal intercourse. It is also possible to transmit the bacteria to a person's eyes if they touch them after being in contact with an infected person's genitals. Oral sex with an infected person can also result in an infection of the throat.[30]

Clinical diagnosis of chlamydia in women is very reliable with a cervical smear. Men can also be tested for chlamydia, which usually involves inserting a swab into the urethra to extract the fluid to be tested. Chlamydia is easily treated with antibiotics prescribed by a doctor. Since it is common for there to not be any symptoms of a chlamydia infection, physicians often screen young women during regular checkups.[31]

Other STIs

In addition to bacterial and viral infections that are sexually transmitted, there are other organisms that can cause infections. Yeast and trichomoniasis are two other such STIs. As with other STIs, clinical diagnosis and regular checkups are important to maintaining sexual health.

Candidiasis (Fungal)

Candida albicans, a yeast-like fungus, causes candidiasis. In a normal vaginal environment, yeast usually do not produce symptoms. However, there can be an overgrowth of naturally occurring yeast if there are changes to the vaginal environment. Antibiotics, birth control pills, IUDs, pregnancy, and diabetes can contribute to altering the vaginal environment and lead to a yeast infection. Poorly ventilated genitals from wearing tight or synthetic clothes can also contribute to developing a yeast infection. Symptoms of a yeast infection include intense itching of the vulva in women, inflammation and soreness of the genitals, and a thick, white, curd-like discharge. Yeast infections also occur in men (the symptoms are similar to what is described above, in the urethral opening and surrounding genital areas), and in the mouth of both men and women.[32]

Candida can be transmitted between partners through vaginal and anal intercourse, as well as during oral sex. However, most yeast infections in women are caused by an imbalance in the vaginal environment and not necessarily through sexual transmission. There are many over-the-counter treatments for yeast infections, including oral, topical, and suppository treatments. You can ask your healthcare provider or your pharmacist more about specific treatments for yeast infections.[33]

Trichomoniasis

Trichomonas vaginalis, a single-celled parasite, causes the most common STI: Trichomoniasis. Symptoms include burning and itching of the vulva, mild pain during intercourse, and an odorous, foamy, whitish to yellowy-greenish discharge, though many women do not exhibit symptoms. In men, there may be tingling or itching in the urethra, though most men do not show symptoms either. The transmission of HIV can be facilitated by a trichomonas infection.[34]

The vast majority of "trich" infections are transmitted through sexual contact. This parasite can survive for several hours in moist environments outside of the body. Contact with infected seminal or vaginal fluids on towels, washcloths, and bedding can transmit this STI. Unlike most STIs, *Trichomonas* can be spread from a toilet seat.[35]

Diagnosis is based on a microscopic examination of vaginal or penile fluids. A treatment of metronidazole can be prescribed for a positive diagnosis.[36]

Breast Exams

Regular breast exams are part of leading a healthy life. Some women schedule monthly self-exams to do while in the shower or as part of their bathroom routine. Adding a reminder to your calendar, or using a period tracking app with a built-in reminder, are excellent ways to integrate this form of self-care into your life. After the age of forty, women should begin having regular breast exams from their doctor in addition to their at-home routine.

Breast cancer is the leading form of cancer among women, but it doesn't affect women alone: men are also susceptible to the disease (although largely after the age of sixty).[37] Eighty percent of lumps found in breast tissue will be benign (non-cancerous), which is good news. Being able to regularly check out your body and being familiar with what your "normal" is will help create a baseline for noticing if things change.

See your health care provider if: you detect a lump or change in the breast, you notice nipple discharge, if you see a "pulling in" of the nipple, or if you perceive a change in the texture, color, or dimpling of the skin.[38]

Now, how to do a self-breast exam! The description below has been used with permission by the Feminist Women's Health Center/Cedar River Clinics.[39]

With breast exams, we are aiming to create a baseline for your body. If you are a human who menstruates, it's better to wait a day or two after your period since around this time of the month breasts tend to be more tender and swollen.

Visual Inspection

Stand in front of a mirror with your upper body unclothed and pressing both hands behind your head.

Look for changes in the shape and size of your breasts.

Check for dimples of the skin or "pulling in" of the nipples.

Check for scaling or a rash on your breasts and nipples.

Next, place your hands on your hips and press firmly inward, tightening your chest muscles, while looking at your breasts for any change in their usual appearance. Perform leaning slightly forward and again while standing upright.

Feeling your Breasts

Circular Method

Please note that there are different techniques for the type of touch used in this part of the examination. For this introduction to a self-exam, I only describe the

Circular Method. For more information, please ask your health provider or refer to the Feminist Women's Health Center/Cedar River Clinics' online resource.

Use the hand opposite the breast you are examining, beginning at the outermost top of your breast.

Press the flat portions of the second, third, and fourth fingertips into your breast.

Move in small circles slowly around your breast, working toward the nipple.

Press gently to feel tissues under the skin and more firmly to feel deep tissues.

Cover all areas of the breast.

Repeat for the opposite breast.

Lying Down

Masses in the lower part of the breast may be more easily felt lying down.

To examine your left breast, lie flat on your back with a pillow or folded towel under your left shoulder.

Raise your left arm over your head.

Use the flat portions of the second, third, and fourth fingertips of your right hand to examine your left breast using the method described previously.

Press gently to feel tissues under the skin and then more firmly for deep tissues.

Repeat for the right breast.

Standing Up

Masses in the upper part of the breast are easier to detect while standing upright.

Place your left hand behind your head, and with the flat portions of the second, third, and fourth fingertips of the right hand, examine your entire left breast using the circular method described.

Repeat for your right breast.

Nipple Area

Gently squeeze your left nipple between your right index finger and thumb and look for any discharge.

Repeat for right nipple.

Additional Areas

Check the area between the upper outer breast and your armpit, as well as the armpit itself.

Check the area just above your collarbones for enlarged lymph nodes.

Breast exams are an excellent way to stay aware of changes in your breasts throughout your life.

Safe Porting

In chapter 9, I mentioned a communication tool called "safe porting." This is a tool that I use often throughout my life: in conversation, when using physical touch, and in sensual situations, to name just a few. Safe porting is a maritime phrase which describes a situation in which a ship can safely enter, use, and then depart from a port without any abnormal occurrences.[40] When I use the term "safe port" I mean that I create a situation for the other person, whether in communicating or in a physical situation, in which they are not surprised at any point.

To create a safe port, you tell someone what you are going to do before you do it. This is an excellent tool to use when having a sensual experience with another person, but it is also useful in many types of situations that don't include sex. For example, if someone has ever startled you before they went in to give you a hug, or brushed up against you in passing as a way of saying hi. These are non-deliberate ways of touching people, and while it has potential for being a good experience, more often than not unexpected-touching or contact creates surprise.

Safe porting can take different forms. You can be direct and simply say "I'm going to touch your arm" or "would you like me to touch your arm?" Give the person the opportunity to accept or reject your offer. Either way it is a win-win: if they want the contact, you can give it to them, and if they don't want the contact, you won't be giving them something they don't want. A safe port could also include more casual offers, like "how about a hug?" Anything where you tell or ask the person what you would like to do *before* you do it acts as a safe port.

If you feel awkward safe porting, you can tell the person you're communicating with that this is a method of communication you're going to use. It may seem strange at first, but that's just because we're not used to being deliberate. All surprise is bad (at first) and by communicating your intention prior to acting, you create a safe and more pleasurable experience for the other person, whether that's your partner in bed or your mom at the dining room table.

WORKS CITED

Introduction: My Fundamentals

Orenstein, Peggy. *Girls & Sex: Navigating the Complicated New Landscape*. Harper, 2016. Page 12.

Chapter 1: Sensuality and Sexuality

"Deliberate, adj." *OED Online*, Oxford University Press, June 2018, www.oed.com /view/Entry/49345. Accessed 25 July 2018.

Gunther, Randi. "Sexy, Sensual or Intimate—What Is Your Sexual Style?" *The Huffington Post*, TheHuffingtonPost.com, 6 Dec. 2017, www.huffingtonpost .com/randi-gunther/sexy-sensual-or-intimate-_b_6582638.html.

Kemp, Kristen. "Uncover Your Sensual Side." *Cosmopolitan*, Cosmopolitan, 14 Nov. 2007, www.cosmopolitan.com/sex-love/advice/a2124/uncover-sensual-side/.

Lew, Alan. *This Is Real and You Are Completely Unprepared: the Days of Awe as a Journey of Transformation*. Back Bay Books/Little, Brown and Company, 2003.

"sensual, adj. and n." *OED Online*, Oxford University Press, June 2018, www.oed.com /view/Entry/176013. Accessed 2 September 2018.

Citations for products with "Sensual" descriptor

"Mandy Synthetic Wig by Sensual." *Wigs Enthusiasts, Hair Extensions and Hairpieces - Best Wig Outlet*, www.bestwigoutlet.com/product/mandy-synthetic-wig-by-sensual .html?gclid=EAIaIQobChMI45_uof-N3AIVkY-zCh1JSw68EAkYCCABEgKaC _D_BwE%2C.

"The Sensual Lip Satin." *Kevyn Aucoin Beauty*, kevynaucoin.com/products/the-sensual -lip-satin?variant=42865597772&gclid=EAIaIQobChMI45_uof-N3AIVkY -zCh1JSw68EAkYASABEgIo2PD_BwE%2C.

"Sensuality Massage & Body Oil 4 Fl Oz (118 ML) Bottle | Piping Rock Health Products." *Piping Rock*, www.pipingrock.com/massage-oils/sensuality-massage -body-oil-7481?prd=D0000J&gclid=EAIaIQobChMI45_uof-N3AIVkY-zCh1 JSw68EAkYAyABEgJ9SvD_BwE%2C%2Bherbal%2Btea-%2Bhttps%3A %2F%2Fnatalydeals.com%2Fproducts%2Fthe-sensual-tea-1sob-10g%29.

Chapter 2: Anatomy with an Emphasis on Pleasure

Ackerman, Diane. *A Natural History of the Senses*. Vintage, 1991.

Balcombe, Jonathan P. *Pleasurable Kingdom: Animals and the Nature of Feeling Good*. Palgrave Macmillan, 2007.

Bolin, Anne, and Patricia Whelehan. *Perspectives on Human Sexuality*. State University of New York Press, 1999.

Corinna, Heather. "Can You Tell Me about Inverted Nipples?" *Scarleteen*, 4 Aug. 2018, www.scarleteen.com/article/advice/can_you_tell_me_about_inverted_nipples.

Corinna, Heather. "Meet Your Prostate!" *Scarleteen*, 22 Jan. 2014, www.scarleteen.com /article/advice/meet_your_prostate.

Corinna, Heather. *S.E.X.: The All-You-Need-to-Know Sexuality Guide to Get You through Your Teens and Twenties*. 2nd ed., Da Capo Lifelong Books, 2016.

Corinna, Heather. "With Pleasure: A View of Whole Sexual Anatomy for Every Body." *Scarleteen*, 19 Apr. 2018, www.scarleteen.com/article/bodies/with _pleasure_a_view_of_whole_sexual_anatomy_for_every_body.

"Cliteracy | Sophia Wallace | TEDxSalford." Performance by Sophia Wallace, *YouTube*, TEDx Talks, 15 July 2015, www.youtube.com/watch?v=dg2RoARuAHM.

"Human Skin." *Britannica Library*, Encyclopædia Britannica, 25 Nov. 2015, library -eb-com.ezproxy.sfpl.org/levels/referencecenter/article/human-skin/106316. Accessed 21 Aug. 2018.

Informed Health Online [Internet]. Cologne, Germany: Institute for Quality and Efficiency in Health Care (IQWiG); 2006. How does the hand work? 2010 Aug 31 [Updated 2016 Dec 23]. Available from: https://www.ncbi.nlm.nih.gov /books/NBK279362/.

Marino, Vincent Di, and Hubert Lepidi. *Anatomic Study of the Clitoris and the Bulbo-Clitoral Organ*. Springer, 2014. Page 81.

Mascall, Sharon. "Time for Rethink on the Clitoris." *BBC News*, BBC, 11 June 2006, news.bbc.co.uk/2/hi/health/5013866.stm.

O'Connell, H., and J. Delancey. "Clitoral Anatomy in Nulliparous, Healthy, Premenopausal Volunteers Using Unenhanced Magnetic Resonance Imaging." *The Journal of Urology*, vol. 173, no. 6, 14 Nov. 2005, pages 2060–2063, doi:10 .1097/01.ju.0000158446.21396.c0.

"Physical Development in Boys: What to Expect." *Healthy Children*, 22 May 2015, www.healthychildren.org/English/ages-stages/gradeschool/puberty/Pages /Physical-Development-Boys-What-to-Expect.aspx.

"Research." *Merriam-Webster.com*. Merriam-Webster, n.d. Web. 20 Aug. 2018.

Reynoso, Hector. "Fingertip Sensory Nerve Endings." *Center for Academic Research and Training in Anthropogeny*, carta.anthropogeny.org/moca/topics/fingertip-sensory -nerve-endings.

Rogers, John. "Testing for and the role of anal and rectal sensation." *Baillière's Clinical Gastroenterology* Volume 6. Issue 1 (1992): Pages 179–191. Science Direct. Web. 5 September 2018 Accessed.

Rose, James D. "The Genital Sensory System." *Sensory Systems II: Senses Other Than Vision*, by Jeremy M. Wolfe, Birkhauser, 1988, pages 24–26.

Schatten, Heide, and Gheorghe M. Constantinescu. *Comparative Reproductive Biology*. John Wiley & Sons, 2008.

Stewart, Elizabeth Gunther, and Paula Spencer. *The V Book: A Doctor's Guide to Complete Vulvovaginal Health*. Bantam Books, 2002.

Szykman, M.; Van Horn, R. C.; Engh, A.L.; Boydston, E. E.; Holekamp, K. E. "Courtship and mating in free-living spotted hyenas" (PDF). *Behaviour*. 16 May 2007.

Chapter 3: Puberty, Bodies, and, Oh, These Changing Times

Arain, Mariam et al. "Maturation of the Adolescent Brain." *Neuropsychiatric Disease and Treatment* 9 (2013): 449–461. PMC. Web. 10 Sept. 2018.

Bailey, K. Alysse, et al. "How Do You Define Body Image? Exploring Conceptual Gaps in Understandings of Body Image at an Exercise Facility." *Body Image*, vol. 23, 23 Dec. 2017, pages 69–79. doi:10.1016/j.bodyim.2017.08.003.

"Body Image." *National Eating Disorders Association*, 22 Feb. 2018, www
.nationaleatingdisorders.org/body-image-0.

Corinna, Heather. *S.E.X.: The All-You-Need-to-Know Progressive Sexuality Guide to Get
You through High School and College*. Da Capo, 2007.

NPR. "'Girls & Sex' and the Importance of Talking to Young Women about Pleasure."
NPR, 29 Mar. 2016, www.npr.org/sections/health-shots/2016/03/29/472211301
/girls-sex-and-the-importance-of-talking-to-young-women-about-pleasure.

Taylor, Sonya Renee. *The Body Is Not an Apology: The Power of Radical Self-Love*.
Berrett-Koehler Publishers, 2018.

Chapter 4: Menarche and Heat Cycles

Menstruation

Corinna, Heather. *S.E.X.: The All-You-Need-to-Know Sexuality Guide to Get You
through Your Teens and Twenties*. 2nd ed., Da Capo Lifelong Books, 2016.

French, Valerie. "A Quick Guide to Skipping Periods with Birth Control." *Bedsider*, 19
Sept. 2013, www.bedsider.org/features/290-a-quick-guide-to-skipping-periods
-with-birth-control.

DeLuca Stein, Robyn. "The Good News about PMS." *TED*, Nov. 2014, www.ted.com
/talks/robyn_stein_deluca_the_good_news_about_pms/details?language=en.

Druet, Anna. "How Did Menstruation Become Taboo?" *Clue*, 7 Sept. 2017, helloclue
.com/articles/culture/how-did-menstruation-become-taboo.

Druet, Anna, and Lisa Kennelly. "Is Period Slang Ever Useful?" *Clue*, 19 Sept. 2017,
helloclue.com/articles/culture/is-period-slang-ever-useful.

Kennelly, Lisa. "The Top Three PMS Myths." *Clue*, 25 Aug. 2015, helloclue.com
/articles/cycle-a-z/top-3-pms-myths.

Kvatum, Lia. "A Period Comes to an End: 100 Years of Menstruation Products." *The
Washington Post*, WP Company, 25 Apr. 2016, www.washingtonpost.com
/national/health-science/a-period-comes-to-an-end-100-years-of-menstruation
-products/2016/04/25/1afe3898-057e-11e6-bdcb-0133da18418d_story.html
?noredirect=on&utm_term=.434cf8260008.

Ironside, Andrew. "Marc Rudov on 'the Downside' of a Woman President." *Media Matters for America*, 11 Mar. 2008, www.mediamatters.org/research/2008/03/11/marc-rudov-on-the-downside-of-a-woman-president/142850.

Moss, Gabrielle. "Six Ways to Make Your Period More Earth-Friendly." *Bustle*, Bustle, 15 Dec. 2015, www.bustle.com/articles/129938-6-ways-to-be-environmentally-conscious-during-your-period.

OWH: Office of Women's Health. U.S. Department of Health & Human Services. March 16, 2018, https://www.womenshealth.gov/a-z-topics/menstruation-and-menstrual-cycle.

Shirozu, H, et al. "Penile Tumescence in the Human Fetus at Term—a Preliminary Report." *U.S. National Library of Medicine*, Early Human Development, 28 Apr. 1995, www.ncbi.nlm.nih.gov/pubmed/7635068.

Thompson, Kirsten MJ. "A Brief History of Birth Control in the U.S." *Our Bodies Ourselves*, 13 Dec. 2013, www.ourbodiesourselves.org/book-excerpts/health-article/a-brief-history-of-birth-control/.

Heat Cycles

Balcombe, Jonathan P. *Pleasurable Kingdom: Animals and the Nature of Feeling Good*. Palgrave Macmillan, 2007.

Mcclintock, Martha K. "Menstrual Synchrony and Suppression." *Nature*, vol. 229, no. 5282, 22 Jan. 1971, doi:10.1038/229244a0.

"Reproductive Behaviour." *Britannica Library*, Encyclopædia Britannica, 10 Aug. 2018, library-eb-com.ezproxy.sfpl.org/levels/referencecenter/article/reproductive-behaviour/110426. Accessed 27 Aug. 2018.

Stewart, Elizabeth Gunther, and Paula Spencer. *The V Book: A Doctor's Guide to Complete Vulvovaginal Health*. Bantam Books, 2002.

Chapter 5: "The M-Thing" and Taking Care of Your Body

Abramson, Paul R. "The Relationship of the Frequency of Masturbation to Several Aspects of Personality and Behavior." *The Journal of Sex Research*. Vol. 9, No. 2. May 1973. pages 132–142.

Eakin, Emily. "BOOKS OF THE TIMES; The Lonely Pleasure, from Sinful to Symbolic." *The New York Times*, The New York Times, 26 Apr. 2003, www .nytimes.com/2003/04/26/books/books-of-the-times-the-lonely-pleasure-from -sinful-to-symbolic.html.

Informed Health Online [Internet]. Cologne, Germany: Institute for Quality and Efficiency in Health Care (IQWiG); 2006. How does the hand work? 2010 Aug 31 [Updated 2016 Dec 23]. Available from: https://www.ncbi.nlm.nih.gov /books/NBK279362/.

Reece, Michael, et al. "National Survey of Sexual Health and Behavior." *Indiana University School of Public Health*, Church & Dwight Co. Inc, 1 Oct. 2010, www.nationalsexstudy.indiana.edu/.

Stewart, Elizabeth Gunther, and Paula Spencer. *The V Book: A Doctor's Guide to Complete Vulvovaginal Health*. Bantam Books, 2002.

Chapter 6: The Big "O"

Blanchflower, David G, and Andrew Oswald. "Unhappiness and Pain in Modern America: A Review Essay, and Further Evidence, on Carol Graham's Happiness for All?" *National Bureau of Economic Research*, University of Chicago Press, Nov. 2017, www.nber.org/papers/w24087.

Blechner, Mark J. "Female Sexual Pleasure." *Psychology Today*, Sussex Publishers, 15 Sept. 2013, www.psychologytoday.com/us/blog/contemporary-psychoanalysis-in -action/201309/female-sexual-pleasure.

Darroch, Jacqueline E., et al. "Differences in Teenage Pregnancy Rates among Five Developed Countries: The Roles of Sexual Activity and Contracep- tive Use." *Guttmacher Institute*, 1 Nov. 2001, www.guttmacher.org/journals /psrh/2001/11/differences-teenage-pregnancy-rates-among-five-developed -countries-roles.

Clark, Mary Pat. "Election, Tragedies Dominate Top Stories of 2012." *Pew Research Center for the People and the Press*, 20 Dec. 2012, www.people-press.org/2012 /12/20/election-tragedies-dominate-top-stories-of-2012/.

Eve Appeal. "Why 'Vagina' Should Be Part of Every Young Woman's Vocabulary," https://eveappeal.org.uk/wp-content/uploads/2016/07/The-Eve-Appeal-Vagina -Dialogues.pdf.

Gusovsky, Dina. "Americans Consume Vast Majority of the World's Opioids." *CNBC*, CNBC, 27 Apr. 2016, www.cnbc.com/2016/04/27/americans-consume-almost -all-of-the-global-opioid-supply.html.

Henderson, Alex. "5 Countries That Do It Better: How Sexual Prudery Makes America a Less Healthy and Happy Place." *Alternet*, 12 Apr. 2012, www.alternet.org /story/154970/5_countries_that_do_it_better:_how_sexual_prudery_makes _america_a_less_healthy_and_happy_place.

Koepsel, Erica R. "The Power in Pleasure: Practical Implementation of Pleasure in Sex Education Classrooms." *American Journal of Sexuality Education*, vol. 11, no. 3, 24 Aug. 2016, pages 205–265, doi:10.1080/15546128.2016.1209451.

Lee, Bruce Y. "50% of Men Don't Know Where the Vagina Is, According to UK Study." *Forbes*, Forbes Magazine, 3 Sept. 2017, www.forbes.com/sites/brucelee /2017/09/03/50-of-men-dont-know-where-the-vagina-is-according-to-uk-study/.

Masters, William, and Virginia E. Johnson. *Human Sexual Response.* Boston: Little, Brown, 1966.

Marino, Vincent Di, and Hubert Lepidi. *Anatomic Study of the Clitoris and the Bulbo-Clitoral Organ.* Springer, 2014. Page 81.

Moalem, Sharon. *How Sex Works: Why We Look, Smell, Taste, Feel, and Act the Way We Do.* HarperCollins, 2009. Page 33.

Nowak, Lynne. "America's Pain Points." *Express Scripts*, 9 Dec. 2014, lab.express -scripts.com/lab/insights/drug-safety-and-abuse/americas-pain-points.

O'Connell, H., and J. Delancey. "Clitoral Anatomy in Nulliparous, Healthy, Premenopausal Volunteers Using Unenhanced Magnetic Resonance Imaging." *The Journal of Urology*, vol. 173, no. 6, 14 Nov. 2005, pages 2060–2063, doi:10.1097/01.ju.0000158446.21396.c0.

"Orgasm." *Oxford English Dictionary.* Third Edition, Updated: September 2004. Accessed: 7 July 2018, http://www.oed.com.ezproxy.sfpl.org/view/Entry/132485 ?rskey=OxgHjZ&result=1&isAdvanced=false#eid.

Stewart, Elizabeth Gunther, and Paula Spencer. *The V Book: A Doctor's Guide to Complete Vulvovaginal Health.* Bantam Books, 2002.

Timmers, Richard L., et al. "Treating Goal-Directed Intimacy." *Social Work*, vol. 21, no. 5, 1976, pages 401–402. *JSTOR*, JSTOR, www.jstor.org/stable/23711841. Page 401.

Chapter 7: How Do You DO?

Becker, Samuel. "Should These Companies Have Their Ads Be Labeled as Too Sexy?" *The Cheat Sheet*, 28 Dec. 2017, www.cheatsheet.com/money-career /hypersexualized-ads-turned-you-off-famous-brands.html/.

Corinna, Heather. *S.E.X.: The All-You-Need-to-Know Progressive Sexuality Guide to Get You through High School and College*. 2nd ed., Da Capo, 2016.

Frederick, David A., et al. "Differences in Orgasm Frequency among Gay, Lesbian, Bisexual, and Heterosexual Men and Women in a U.S. National Sample." *Archives of Sexual Behavior*, vol. 47, no. 1, 2017, pages 273–288, doi:10.1007 /s10508-017-0939-z.

Kinnaman, David, and Roxy Lee Stone. "Porn in the Digital Age: New Research Reveals 10 Trends." *Barna Group*, 6 Apr. 2016, www.barna.com/research/porn -in-the-digital-age-new-research-reveals-10-trends/.

Lucke, Jayne. "Sex, Health and Society: What's the Connection?" *The Conversation*, 24 May 2015, theconversation.com/sex-health-and-society-whats-the-connection -42191.

O'Hara, Ross E., et al. "Greater Exposure to Sexual Content in Popular Movies Predicts Earlier Sexual Debut and Increased Sexual Risk Taking." *NCBI*, U.S. National Library of Medicine, 1 Sept. 2012, www.ncbi.nlm.nih.gov/pmc/articles /PMC3779897/.

Sellgren, Katherine. "Pornography 'Desensitising Young People'." *BBC News*, BBC, 15 June 2016, www.bbc.com/news/education-36527681.

"Sex, n.1." *OED Online*, Oxford University Press, June 2018, www.oed.com/view /Entry/176989. Accessed 12 August 2018.

Sobecki, Janelle N., et al. "What We Don't Talk about When We Don't Talk about Sex: Results of a National Survey of U.S. Obstetrician/Gynecologists." *The Journal of Sexual Medicine*, vol. 9, no. 5, May 2012, pages 1285–1294, doi:10.1111 /j.1743-6109.2012.02702.x.

Timmers, Richard L., et al. "Treating Goal-Directed Intimacy." *Social Work*, vol. 21, no. 5, 1976, pages 401–402. *JSTOR*, JSTOR, www.jstor.org/stable/23711841. Page 401.

Chapter 8: Safe Sex and All about Latex

C., Anna. "STD Awareness: Can I Use Plastic Wrap as a Dental Dam During Oral Sex?" *Planned Parenthood Advocates of Arizona*, 4 Jan. 2016, advocatesazorg/2016 /01/04/std-awareness-can-i-use-plastic-wrap-as-a-dental-dam-during-oral-sex/.

Corinna, Heather. "Honorably Discharged: A Guide to Vaginal Secretions." *Scarleteen*, 4 May 2018, www.scarleteen.com/article/bodies/honorably_discharged_a_guide _to_vaginal_secretions.

Corinna, Heather. *S.E.X.: The All-You-Need-to-Know Progressive Sexuality Guide to Get You through High School and College*. 2nd ed., Da Capo, 2016. Pages 285–300.

Corinna, Heather. "What's That Fluid?" *Scarleteen*, 12 June 2018, www.scarleteen .com/article/advice/whats_that_fluid.

Jozkowski, Kristen N., et al. "Women's Perceptions about Lubricant Use and Vaginal Wetness during Sexual Activities." Wiley Online Library, *The Journal of Sexual Medicine*, 4 Dec. 2012, onlinelibrary.wiley.com/doi/abs/10.1111/jsm.12022 ?deniedAccessCustomisedMessage=.

Reece, Michael, et al. "Men's Use and Perceptions of Commercial Lubricants: Prevalence and Characteristics in a Nationally Representative Sample of American Adults." Wiley Online Library, *The Journal of Sexual Medicine*, 26 Feb. 2014, onlinelibrary.wiley.com/doi/abs/10.1111/jsm.12480.

Stewart, Elizabeth Gunther, and Paula Spencer. *The V Book: A Doctor's Guide to Complete Vulvovaginal Health*. Bantam Books, 2002.

Lindberg, Laura Duberstein, and Isaac Maddow-Zimet. "Consequences of Sex Education on Teen and Young Adult Sexual Behaviors and Outcomes." *Journal of Adolescent Health*, vol. 51, no. 4, Oct. 2012, pages 332–338, doi:10.1016/j .jadohealth.2011.12.028.

O'Hara, Ross E., et al. "Greater Exposure to Sexual Content in Popular Movies Predicts Earlier Sexual Debut and Increased Sexual Risk Taking." *NCBI*, U.S. National Library of Medicine, 1 Sept. 2012, www.ncbi.nlm.nih.gov/pmc/articles /PMC3779897/.

"What You Need to Know about . . . Personal Lubricants." *AASECT*, www.aasect.org /what-you-need-know-about-personal-lubricants.

Chapter 9: Double "C's"—Communication and Consent

Corinna, Heather. "Driver's Ed for the Sexual Superhighway: Navigating Consent." *Scarleteen*, 13 May 2016, www.scarleteen.com/article/abuse_assault/drivers_ed _for_the_sexual_superhighway_navigating_consent. Accessed 10 July 2018.

"Understanding Consent." *About RAINN | RAINN*, rainn.org/understanding-consent. Accessed 10 July 2018.

"What Is Sexual Consent? | Facts About Rape & Sexual Assault." *Planned Parenthood*, National-PPFA, www.plannedparenthood.org/learn/sex-and-relationships/sexual -consent. Accessed 10 July 2018.

Chapter 10: The Nuts and Bolts of Friendship

"friend." American Heritage® Dictionary of the English Language, Fifth Edition. 2011. Houghton Mifflin Harcourt Publishing Company 31 Jul. 2018. https://www .thefreedictionary.com/friend.

Chapter 11: How to Talk about the Birds and the Bees

American Adolescents' Sources of Sexual Health Information." *Guttmacher Institute*, 21 Dec. 2017, www.guttmacher.org/fact-sheet/facts-american-teens-sources -information-about-sex.

Knowles, Jon. *Sex Education in the United States*. Issue Brief. Planned Parenthood Federation of America, Inc., March 2012.

Martino, Steven C, et al. "Beyond the 'Big Talk': The Roles of Breadth and Repetition in Parent-Adolescent Communication about Sexual Topics." *AAP News and Journals Gateway*, Pediatrics, Mar. 2008, VOLUME 121 / ISSUE 3, http:// pediatrics.aappublications.org/content/121/3/e612.

Orenstein, Peggy. *Girls & Sex: Navigating the Complicated New Landscape*. Harper, 2016.

Willinsky, John. "Chapter 8: Learning the Language of Difference: The Dictionary in the High School." *Counterpoints*, vol. 184, 2001, pages 171–185. *JSTOR*, JSTOR, www.jstor.org/stable/42976661.

Resources for Continued Education

"Birth Control Methods." *Bedsider*, Power to Decide, www.bedsider.org/methods.

"Hepatitis C Questions and Answers for the Public." *Centers for Disease Control and Prevention*, 12 June 2018, www.cdc.gov/hepatitis/hcv/cfaq.htm.

"HPV and Men: CDC Fact Sheet." *Centers for Disease Control and Prevention*, 14 July 2017, www.cdc.gov/std/hpv/stdfact-hpv-and-men.htm.

"Male Breast Cancer." *MedlinePlus*, U.S. National Library of Medicine, 23 Aug. 2018, medlineplus.gov/malebreastcancer.html.

Punukollu, M. "Self Breast Exam." *Women's Health Information*, Feminist Women's Health Center, 2011, www.fwhc.org/health/self-breast-exam.htm.

Steamship Mutual. Sea Venture Vol. 18, June 1999. Accessed on 22 August 2017, https://www.steamshipmutual.com/publications/Articles/Articles/Safe_Port.asp.

Singh, Neeta. "HPV and Cervical Cancer." *Cancer Research*, American Association for Cancer Research, 1 May 2008, cancerres.aacrjournals.org/content/68/9_Supplement/4717.short.

Wald, Anna. "Investigational HPV Vaccine Shows 100% Efficacy." *NEJM Journal Watch*, 22 Nov. 2005, www.jwatch.org/wh200511220000001/2005/11/22/investigational-hpv-vaccine-shows-100-efficacy.

NOTES

Introduction

1.   Knowles, Jon. *Sex Education in the United States*. Issue Brief. Planned Parenthood
      Federation of America, Inc., March 2012.

2.   "American Adolescents' Sources of Sexual Health Information." *Guttmacher
      Institute*, 21 Dec. 2017, www.guttmacher.org/fact-sheet/facts-american-teens
      -sources-information-about-sex.

3.   Koepsel, Erica R. "The Power in Pleasure: Practical Implementation of Pleasure
      in Sex Education Classrooms." *American Journal of Sexuality Education*, vol. 11,
      no. 3, 24 Aug. 2016, pp. 205–265, doi:10.1080/15546128.2016.1209451.

4.   Knowles, Jon. *Sex Education in the United States*. Issue Brief. Planned Parenthood
      Federation of America, Inc., March 2012. Page 2.

5.   Orgasm Frequency among Gay, Lesbian, Bisexual, and Heterosexual Men and
      Women in a U.S. National Sample." *Archives of Sexual Behavior*, vol. 47, no. 1,
      2017, pp. 273–288, doi:10.1007/s10508-017-0939-z.

6.   "Victims of Sexual Violence: Statistics." *RAINN*, www.rainn.org/statistics
      /victims-sexual-violence.

7.   Orenstein, Peggy. *Girls & Sex: Navigating the Complicated New Landscape*.
      Harper, 2016. Page 12.

Chapter 1

1.   "Sensual, adj. and n." *OED Online*, Oxford University Press, June 2018, www
      .oed.com/view/Entry/176013. Accessed 2 September 2018.

2.   Gunther, Randi. "Sexy, Sensual or Intimate—What Is Your Sexual Style?" *The
      Huffington Post*, TheHuffingtonPost.com, 6 Dec. 2017, www.huffingtonpost
      .com/randi-gunther/sexy-sensual-or-intimate-_b_6582638.html.

3. Kemp, Kristen. "Uncover Your Sensual Side." *Cosmopolitan*, Cosmopolitan, 14 Nov. 2007, www.cosmopolitan.com/sex-love/advice/a2124/uncover-sensual -side/.

4. "The Sensual Lip Satin." *Kevyn Aucoin Beauty*, kevynaucoin.com/products/the -sensual-lip-satin?variant=42865597772&gclid=EAIaIQobChMI45_uof -N3AIVkY-zCh1JSw68EAkYASABEgIo2PD_BwE%2C.

5. "Mandy Synthetic Wig by Sensual." *Wigs Enthusiasts, Hair Extensions and Hairpieces-Best Wig Outlet*, www.bestwigoutlet.com/product/mandy-synthetic -wig-by-sensual.html?gclid=EAIaIQobChMI45_uof-N3AIVkY -zCh1JSw68EAkYCCABEgKaC_D_BwE%2C.

6. "Sensuality Massage & Body Oil 4 Fl Oz (118 ML) Bottle | Piping Rock Health Products." *Piping Rock*, www.pipingrock.com/massage-oils/sensuality-massage -body-oil-7481?prd=D0000J&gclid=EAIaIQobChMI45_uof-N3AIVkY-zCh1 JSw68EAkYAyABEgJ9SvD_BwE%2C%2Bherbal%2Btea-%2Bhttps%3A%2F %2Fnatalydeals.com%2Fproducts%2Fthe-sensual-tea-1sob-10g%29.

7. "Deliberate, adj." *OED Online*, Oxford University Press, June 2018, www.oed .com/view/Entry/49345. Accessed 25 July 2018.

Part 1
Chapter 2

1. Corinna, Heather. "With Pleasure: A View of Whole Sexual Anatomy for Every Body." *Scarleteen*, 19 Apr. 2018, www.scarleteen.com/article/bodies/with _pleasure_a_view_of_whole_sexual_anatomy_for_every_body.

2. "Human Skin." *Britannica Library*, Encyclopædia Britannica, 25 Nov. 2015, library-eb-com.ezproxy.sfpl.org/levels/referencecenter/article/human-skin /106316. Accessed 21 Aug. 2018.

3. Ackerman, Diane. *A Natural History of the Senses*. Vintage, 1991. Page 68.

4. Ackerman, Diane. *A Natural History of the Senses*. Vintage, 1991. Page 87.

5. Ackerman, Diane. *A Natural History of the Senses*. Vintage, 1991. Page 132.

6. Corinna, "With Pleasure."

7. Informed Health Online. Cologne, Germany: Institute for Quality and Efficiency in Health Care (IQWiG); 2006. How does the hand work? 2010

Aug. 31 [Updated 2016 Dec. 23], https://www.ncbi.nlm.nih.gov/books /NBK279362/.

8.   Reynoso, Hector. "Fingertip Sensory Nerve Endings." *Center for Academic Research and Training in Anthropogeny*, carta.anthropogeny.org/moca/topics /fingertip-sensory-nerve-endings.

9.   Corinna, Heather. *S.E.X.: The All-You-Need-to-Know Sexuality Guide to Get You through Your Teens and Twenties.* 2nd ed., Da Capo Lifelong Books, 2016. Page 22.

10.   Corinna, *S.E.X.* Page 39.

11.   "Physical Development in Boys: What to Expect." *Healthy Children*, 22 May 2015, www.healthychildren.org/English/ages-stages/gradeschool/puberty/Pages /Physical-Development-Boys-What-to-Expect.aspx.

12.   Corinna, Heather. "Can You Tell Me about Inverted Nipples?" *Scarleteen*, 4 Aug. 2018, www.scarleteen.com/article/advice/can_you_tell_me_about_inverted _nipples.

13.   Corinna, "With Pleasure."

14.   Corinna, "With Pleasure."

15.   Corinna, "With Pleasure."

16.   http://www.scarleteen.com/article/advice/giveem_some_lip_labia_that_clearly _aint_minor.

17.   https://dodsonandross.com/index.php/blogs/carlin/2010/05/bettys-vulva -illustrations.

18.   Balcombe, Jonathan P. *Pleasurable Kingdom: Animals and the Nature of Feeling Good.* Palgrave Macmillan, 2007. Page 111.

19.   Szykman, M.; Van Horn, R. C.; Engh, A.L.; Boydston, E. E.; Holekamp, K. E. "Courtship and mating in free-living spotted hyenas" (PDF). *Behaviour.* 16 May 2007. Page 816.

20.   Mascall, Sharon. "Time for Rethink on the Clitoris." *BBC News*, BBC, 11 June 2006, news.bbc.co.uk/2/hi/health/5013866.stm.

21.   O'Connell, H., and J. Delancey. "Clitoral Anatomy in Nulliparous, Healthy, Premenopausal Volunteers Using Unenhanced Magnetic Resonance Imaging." *The Journal of Urology*, vol. 173, no. 6, 14 Nov. 2005, pp. 2060–2063, doi:10 .1097/01.ju.0000158446.21396.c0.

22. O'Connell, "Clitoral Anatomy . . ."

23. Marino, Vincent Di, and Hubert Lepidi. *Anatomic Study of the Clitoris and the Bulbo-Clitoral Organ.* Springer, 2014. Page 81.

24. M., MS. "The Internal Clitoris." Center for Erotic Intelligence. Accessed December 14, 2018, http://centerforeroticintelligence.org/internal-clitoris/.

25. Rose, James D. "The Genital Sensory System." *Sensory Systems II: Senses Other Than Vision*, by Jeremy M. Wolfe, Birkhauser, 1988, pp. 24–26.

26. Corinna, *S.E.X.* Pages 41–45.

27. Corinna, *S.E.X.* Pages 41–45.

28. Corinna, *S.E.X.* Pages 41–45.

29. Corinna, *S.E.X.* Pages 41–45.

30. Schatten, Heide, and Gheorghe M. Constantinescu. *Comparative Reproductive Biology.* John Wiley & Sons, 2008. Pages 9–16.

31. Rogers, John. "Testing for and the role of anal and rectal sensation." *Baillière's Clinical Gastroenterology* Volume 6. Issue 1 (1992): Pages 179-191. Science Direct. Web. 5 September 2018 Accessed.

32. Corinna, "With Pleasure."

33. Corinna, Heather. "Meet Your Prostate!" *Scarleteen*, 22 Jan. 2014, www .scarleteen.com/article/advice/meet_your_prostate.

34. "Cliteracy, Sophia Wallace, TEDxSalford." Performance by Sophia Wallace, *YouTube*, TEDx Talks, 15 July 2015, www.youtube.com/watch?v=dg2 RoARuAHM.

35. Corinna, *S.E.X.* Page 48.

36. Corinna, *S.E.X.* Page 48.

37. Bolin, Anne, and Patricia Whelehan. *Perspectives on Human Sexuality.* State University of New York Press, 1999.

Chapter 3

1. Corinna, *S.E.X.* Page 47.

2. Arain, Mariam et al. "Maturation of the Adolescent Brain." *Neuropsychiatric Disease and Treatment* 9 (2013): 449–461. *PMC.* Web. 10 Sept. 2018.

3. Corinna, Heather. *S.E.X.* Pages 20-3.

4. Corinna, Heather. *S.E.X.* Pages 20-3.

5.   Corinna, Heather. *S.E.X.* Pages 20–3.

6.   Corinna, Heather. *S.E.X.* Pages 20–3.

7.   Corinna, Heather. *S.E.X.* Page 57.

8.   "Bsody Image." *National Eating Disorders Association*, 22 Feb. 2018, www .nationaleatingdisorders.org/body-image-0.

9.   Bailey, K. Alysse, et al. "How Do You Define Body Image? Exploring Conceptual Gaps in Understandings of Body Image at an Exercise Facility." *Body Image*, vol. 23, 23 Dec. 2017, pp. 69–79, doi:10.1016/j.bodyim.2017.08.003.

10. Taylor, Sonya Renee. *The Body Is Not an Apology: The Power of Radical Self-Love.* Berrett-Koehler Publishers, 2018. Page 4.

11. NPR. "'Girls & Sex' and the Importance of Talking to Young Women about Pleasure." *NPR*, 29 Mar. 2016, www.npr.org/sections/health-shots/2016/03/29 /472211301/girls-sex-and-the-importance-of-talking-to-young-women-about -pleasure.

12. NPR. "'Girls & Sex'."

Chapter 4

1.   Druet, Anna, and Lisa Kennelly. "Is Period Slang Ever Useful?" *Clue*, 19 Sept. 2017, helloclue.com/articles/culture/is-period-slang-ever-useful.

2.   Kennelly, Lisa. "The Top Three PMS Myths." *Clue*, 25 Aug. 2015, helloclue .com/articles/cycle-a-z/top-3-pms-myths.

3.   Druet, Anna. "How Did Menstruation Become Taboo?" *Clue*, 7 Sept. 2017, helloclue.com/articles/culture/how-did-menstruation-become-taboo.

4.   DeLuca Stein, Robyn. "The Good News about PMS." *TED*, Nov. 2014, www .ted.com/talks/robyn_stein_deluca_the_good_news_about_pms/details ?language=en.

5.   DeLuca Stein, "The Good News about PMS." *TED*.

6.   Ironside, Andrew. "Marc Rudov on 'the Downside' of a Woman President." *Media Matters for America*, 11 Mar. 2008, www.mediamatters.org/research/2008 /03/11/marc-rudov-on-the-downside-of-a-woman-president/142850.

7.   Corinna, Heather. *S.E.X.* Pages 32–8.

8. OWH: Office of Women's Health. U.S. Department of Health & Human Services. March 16, 2018, https://www.womenshealth.gov/a-z-topics/menstruation -and-menstrual-cycle.

9. Corinna, Heather. *S.E.X.* Page 32.

10. OWH: Office of Women's Health.

11. Corinna, Heather. *S.E.X.* Pages 32–8.

12. Corinna, Heather. *S.E.X.* Page 33.

13. Corinna, Heather. *S.E.X.* Page 45.

14. Shirozu, H, et al. "Penile Tumescence in the Human Fetus at Term—a Preliminary Report." *U.S. National Library of Medicine*, Early Human Development, 28 Apr. 1995, www.ncbi.nlm.nih.gov/pubmed/7635068.

15. Corinna, Heather. *S.E.X.* Pages 41–46.

16. OWH: Office of Women's Health.

17. Corinna, Heather. *S.E.X.* Pages 32–8.

18. Corinna, Heather. *S.E.X.* Pages 32–8.

19. Corinna, Heather. *S.E.X.* Page 38.

20. Kvatum, Lia. "A Period Comes to an End: 100 Years of Menstruation Products." *The Washington Post*, WP Company, 25 Apr. 2016, www.washingtonpost.com /national/health-science/a-period-comes-to-an-end-100-years-of-menstruation -products/2016/04/25/1afe3898-057e-11e6-bdcb-0133da18418d_story.html ?noredirect=on&utm_term=.434cf8260008.

21. Thompson, Kirsten MJ. "A Brief History of Birth Control in the U.S." *Our Bodies Ourselves*, 13 Dec. 2013, www.ourbodiesourselves.org/book-excerpts /health-article/a-brief-history-of-birth-control/.

22. French, Valerie. "A Quick Guide to Skipping Periods with Birth Control." *Bedsider*, 19 Sept. 2013, www.bedsider.org/features/290-a-quick-guide-to-skipping -periods-with-birth-control.

23. Moss, Gabrielle. "Six Ways to Make Your Period More Earth-Friendly." *Bustle*, Bustle, 15 Dec. 2015, www.bustle.com/articles/129938-6-ways-to-be -environmentally-conscious-during-your-period.

24. "Reproductive Behaviour." *Britannica Library*, Encyclopædia Britannica, 10 Aug. 2018, library-eb-com.ezproxy.sfpl.org/levels/referencecenter/article /reproductive-behaviour/110426. Accessed 27 Aug. 2018.

25.   "Reproductive Behaviour." *Britannica Library*, Encyclopædia Britannica, 10 Aug. 2018, library-eb-com.ezproxy.sfpl.org/levels/referencecenter/article/reproductive -behaviour/110426. Accessed 27 Aug. 2018.

26.   Mcclintock, Martha K. "Menstrual Synchrony and Suppression." *Nature*, vol. 229, no. 5282, 22 Jan. 1971, doi:10.1038/229244a0.

27.   Stewart, Elizabeth Gunther, and Paula Spencer. *The V Book: A Doctor's Guide to Complete Vulvovaginal Health*. Bantam Books, 2002. Page 110.

28.   Balcombe, Jonathan P. *Pleasurable Kingdom: Animals and the Nature of Feeling Good*. Palgrave Macmillan, 2007.

Part 2
Chapter 5

1.   Eakin, Emily. "BOOKS OF THE TIMES; The Lonely Pleasure, from Sinful to Symbolic." *The New York Times*, The New York Times, 26 Apr. 2003, www .nytimes.com/2003/04/26/books/books-of-the-times-the-lonely-pleasure-from -sinful-to-symbolic.html.

2.   Patton, Michael S. "Masturbation from Judaism to Victorianism." *Journal of Religion and Health* 24, no. 2 (1985): 133-46, http://www.jstor.org/stable /27505821. Page 134.

3.   Reece, Michael, et al. "National Survey of Sexual Health and Behavior." *Indiana University School of Public Health*, Church & Dwight Co. Inc, 1 Oct. 2010, www.nationalsexstudy.indiana.edu/.

4.   Reece, "National Survery of Sexual Health . . ."

5.   Abramson, Paul R. "The Relationship of the Frequency of Masturbation to Several Aspects of Personality and Behavior." *The Journal of Sex Research*. Vol. 9, No. 2. May 1973. pp. 132-142.

6.   Informed Health Online [Internet]. Cologne, Germany: Institute for Quality and Efficiency in Health Care (IQWiG); 2006. How does the hand work? 2010 Aug. 31 [Updated 2016 Dec. 23], Available from: https://www.ncbi.nlm.nih .gov/books/NBK279362/.

7.   Stewart, Elizabeth Gunther, and Paula Spencer. *The V Book: A Doctor's Guide to Complete Vulvovaginal Health*. Bantam Books, 2002. Page 121.

Chapter 6

1.   Henderson, Alex. "5 Countries That Do It Better: How Sexual Prudery Makes America a Less Healthy and Happy Place." *Alternet*, 12 Apr. 2012, www.alternet. org/story/154970/5_countries_that_do_it_better:_how_sexual_prudery_makes _america_a_less_healthy_and_happy_place.

2.   Koepsel, Erica R. "The Power in Pleasure: Practical Implementation of Pleasure in Sex Education Classrooms." *American Journal of Sexuality Education*, vol. 11, no. 3, 24 Aug. 2016, pp. 205–265, doi:10.1080/15546128.2016.1209451.

3.   Darroch, Jacqueline E., et al. "Differences in Teenage Pregnancy Rates among Five Developed Countries: The Roles of Sexual Activity and Contraceptive Use." *Guttmacher Institute*, 1 Nov. 2001, www.guttmacher.org/journals/psrh/2001/11 /differences-teenage-pregnancy-rates-among-five-developed-countries-roles.

4.   Eve Appeal. "Why 'Vagina' Should Be Part of Every Young Woman's Vocabulary," https://eveappeal.org.uk/wp-content/uploads/2016/07/The-Eve -Appea-Vagina-Dialogues.pdf.

5.   Lee, Bruce Y. "50% of Men Don't Know Where the Vagina Is, According to UK Study." *Forbes*, Forbes Magazine, 3 Sept. 2017, www.forbes.com/sites/brucelee /2017/09/03/50-of-men-dont-know-where-the-vagina-is-according-to-uk-study/.

6.   Clark, Mary Pat. "Election, Tragedies Dominate Top Stories of 2012." *Pew Research Center for the People and the Press*, 20 Dec. 2012, www.people-press .org/2012/12/20/election-tragedies-dominate-top-stories-of-2012/.

7.   Blanchflower, David G, and Andrew Oswald. "Unhappiness and Pain in Modern America: A Review Essay, and Further Evidence, on Carol Graham's Happiness for All?" *National Bureau of Economic Research*, University of Chicago Press, Nov. 2017, www.nber.org/papers/w24087.

8.   Gusovsky, Dina. "Americans Consume Vast Majority of the World's Opioids." *CNBC*, CNBC, 27 Apr. 2016, www.cnbc.com/2016/04/27/americans-consume -almost-all-of-the-global-opioid-supply.html.

9.   Nowak, Lynne. "America's Pain Points." *Express Scripts*, 9 Dec. 2014, lab.express -scripts.com/lab/insights/drug-safety-and-abuse/americas-pain-points.

10. Blechner, Mark J. "Female Sexual Pleasure." *Psychology Today*, Sussex Publishers, 15 Sept. 2013, www.psychologytoday.com/us/blog/contemporary-psychoanalysis -in-action/201309/female-sexual-pleasure.

11. Marino, Vincent Di, and Hubert Lepidi. *Anatomic Study of the Clitoris and the Bulbo-Clitoral Organ*. Springer, 2014. Page 81.

12. O'Connell, H., and J. Delancey. "Clitoral Anatomy in Nulliparous, Healthy, Premenopausal Volunteers Using Unenhanced Magnetic Resonance Imaging." *The Journal of Urology*, vol. 173, no. 6, 14 Nov. 2005, pp. 2060–2063, doi:10 .1097/01.ju.0000158446.21396.c0.

13. Masters, William, and Virginia E. Johnson. *Human Sexual Response*. Boston: Little, Brown, 1966.

14. Stewart, Elizabeth Gunther, and Paula Spencer. *The V Book: A Doctor's Guide to Complete Vulvovaginal Health*. Bantam Books, 2002. Page 111.

15. Timmers, Richard L., et al. "Treating Goal-Directed Intimacy." *Social Work*, vol. 21, no. 5, 1976, pp. 401–402. *JSTOR*, JSTOR, www.jstor.org/stable/23711841. Page 401.

16. "Orgasm." *Oxford English Dictionary*. Third Edition, Updated: September 2004. Accessed: 7 July 2018, http://www.oed.com.ezproxy.sfpl.org/view/Entry/132485 ?rskey=OxgHjZ&result=1&isAdvanced=false#eid.

17. "Orgasm." *Oxford English Dictionary*.

18. Moalem, Sharon. *How Sex Works: Why We Look, Smell, Taste, Feel, and Act the Way We Do*. HarperCollins, 2009. Page 33.

19. Moalem, Sharon. *How Sex Works: Why We Look, Smell, Taste, Feel, and Act the Way We Do*. Harper Collins, 2009. Page 33.

Chapter 7

1. Corinna, Heather. *S.E.X.* Page 182.

2. Corinna, Heather. *S.E.X.* Page 183.

3. Timmers, Richard L., et al. "Treating Goal-Directed Intimacy." *Social Work*, vol. 21, no. 5, 1976, pp. 401–402. *JSTOR*, JSTOR, www.jstor.org/stable/23711841. Page 401.

4. Becker, Samuel. "Should These Companies Have Their Ads Be Labeled as Too Sexy?" *The Cheat Sheet*, 28 Dec. 2017, www.cheatsheet.com/money-career /hypersexualized-ads-turned-you-off-famous-brands.html/.

5. Lucke, Jayne. "Sex, Health and Society: What's the Connection?" *The Conversation*, 24 May 2015, theconversation.com/sex-health-and-society-whats-the-connection-42191.

6. O'Hara, Ross E., et al. "Greater Exposure to Sexual Content in Popular Movies Predicts Earlier Sexual Debut and Increased Sexual Risk Taking." *NCBI*, U.S. National Library of Medicine, 1 Sept. 2012, www.ncbi.nlm.nih.gov/pmc/articles/PMC3779897/.

7. Sellgren, Katherine. "Pornography 'Desensitising Young People'." *BBC News*, BBC, 15 June 2016, www.bbc.com/news/education-36527681.

8. Kinnaman, David, and Roxy Lee Stone. "Porn in the Digital Age: New Research Reveals 10 Trends." *Barna Group*, 6 Apr. 2016, www.barna.com/research/porn-in-the-digital-age-new-research-reveals-10-trends/.

9. O'Hara, "Greater Exposure to Sexual Content."

10. Sobecki, Janelle N., et al. "What We Don't Talk about When We Don't Talk about Sex: Results of a National Survey of U.S. Obstetrician/Gynecologists." *The Journal of Sexual Medicine*, vol. 9, no. 5, May 2012, pages 1285–1294, doi:10.1111/j.1743-6109.2012.02702.x.

11. Frederick, David A., et al. "Differences in Orgasm Frequency among Gay, Lesbian, Bisexual, and Heterosexual Men and Women in a U.S. National Sample." *Archives of Sexual Behavior*, vol. 47, no. 1, 2017, pages 273–288, doi:10.1007/s10508-017-0939-z.

Chapter 8

1. Lindberg, Laura Duberstein, and Isaac Maddow-Zimet. "Consequences of Sex Education on Teen and Young Adult Sexual Behaviors and Outcomes." *Journal of Adolescent Health*, vol. 51, no. 4, Oct. 2012, pages 332–338, doi:10.1016/j.jadohealth.2011.12.028.

2. O'Hara, Ross E., et al. "Greater Exposure to Sexual Content in Popular Movies Predicts Earlier Sexual Debut and Increased Sexual Risk Taking." *NCBI*, U.S. National Library of Medicine, 1 Sept. 2012, www.ncbi.nlm.nih.gov/pmc/articles/PMC3779897/.

3. Corinna, Heather. *S.E.X.* Page 302.

4. Corinna, Heather. *S.E.X.* Page 285.

5.   Stewart, Elizabeth Gunther, and Paula Spencer. *The V Book: A Doctor's Guide to Complete Vulvovaginal Health.* Bantam Books, 2002. Page 126.

6.   Corinna, Heather. *S.E.X.* Page 287.

7.   Corinna, Heather. *S.E.X.* Pages 287–293.

8.   Corinna, Heather. *S.E.X.* Pages 287–293.

9.   Corinna, Heather. *S.E.X.* Pages 287–293.

10. C., Anna. "STD Awareness: Can I Use Plastic Wrap as a Dental Dam During Oral Sex?" *Planned Parenthood Advocates of Arizona*, 4 Jan. 2016, advocatesaz.org /2016/01/04/std-awareness-can-i-use-plastic-wrap-as-a-dental-dam-during -oral-sex/.

11. Reece, Michael, et al. "Men's Use and Perceptions of Commercial Lubricants: Prevalence and Characteristics in a Nationally Representative Sample of American Adults." *Wiley Online Library, The Journal of Sexual Medicine*, 26 Feb. 2014, onlinelibrary.wiley.com/doi/abs/10.1111/jsm.12480.; Jozkowski, Kristen N., et al. "Women's Perceptions about Lubricant Use and Vaginal Wetness during Sexual Activities." Wiley Online Library, *The Journal of Sexual Medicine*, 4 Dec. 2012, onlinelibrary.wiley.com/doi/abs/10.1111/jsm.12022 ?deniedAccessCustomisedMessage=.

12. "What You Need to Know about . . . Personal Lubricants." *AASECT*, www .aasect.org/what-you-need-know-about-personal-lubricants.

13. Corinna, Heather. *S.E.X.* Page 45.

14. Corinna, Heather. "Honorably Discharged: A Guide to Vaginal Secretions." *Scarleteen*, 4 May 2018, www.scarleteen.com/article/bodies/honorably_discharged _a_guide_to_vaginal_secretions.

15. Corinna, Heather. *S.E.X.* Page 45.

16. Stewart, Elizabeth Gunther, and Paula Spencer. *The V Book.* Pages 101–3.

17. Corinna, Heather. "Honorably Discharged."

18. Corinna, Heather. *S.E.X.* Page 45.

19. Corinna, Heather. "What's That Fluid?" *Scarleteen*, 12 June 2018, www .scarleteen.com/article/advice/whats_that_fluid.

20. Stewart, Elizabeth Gunther, and Paula Spencer. *The V Book.* Page 82.

21. Stewart, Elizabeth Gunther, and Paula Spencer. *The V Book.* Page 101.

Part 3

Chapter 9

1. "Understanding Consent." *About RAINN | RAINN*, rainn.org/understanding -consent. Accessed 10 July 2018.

2. "What Is Sexual Consent? | Facts About Rape & Sexual Assault." *Planned Parenthood*, National - PPFA, www.plannedparenthood.org/learn/sex-and-relationships /sexual-consent. Accessed 10 July 2018.

3. Corinna, Heather. "Driver's Ed for the Sexual Superhighway: Navigating Consent." *Scarleteen*, 13 May 2016, www.scarleteen.com/article/abuse_assault /drivers_ed_for_the_sexual_superhighway_navigating_consent. Accessed 10 July 2018.

4. "What Is Sexual Consent? | Facts About Rape & Sexual Assault." *Planned Parenthood*, National - PPFA, www.plannedparenthood.org/learn/sex-and-relationships /sexual-consent. Accessed 10 July 2018.

5. Corinna, Heather. "Driver's Ed for the Sexual Superhighway: Navigating Consent." *Scarleteen*, 13 May 2016, www.scarleteen.com/article/abuse_assault /drivers_ed_for_the_sexual_superhighway_navigating_consent. Accessed 10 July 2018.

Chapter 10

1. "Friend." American Heritage® Dictionary of the English Language, Fifth Edition. 2011. Houghton Mifflin Harcourt Publishing Company 31 July 2018. https:// www.thefreedictionary.com/friend.

Chapter 11

1. Knowles, Jon. *Sex Education in the United States*. Issue Brief. Planned Parenthood Federation of America, Inc., March 2012.

2. "American Adolescents' Sources of Sexual Health Information." *Guttmacher Institute*, 21 Dec. 2017, www.guttmacher.org/fact-sheet/facts-american-teens -sources-information-about-sex.

3. Martino, Steven C, et al. "Beyond the 'Big Talk': The Roles of Breadth and Repetition in Parent-Adolescent Communication about Sexual Topics." *AAP*

News and Journals Gateway, Pediatrics, Mar. 2008, VOLUME 121 / ISSUE 3 http://pediatrics.aappublications.org/content/121/3/e612.

4. Orenstein, Peggy. *Girls & Sex: Navigating the Complicated New Landscape.* Harper, 2016.

5. Willinsky, John. "Chapter 8: Learning the Language of Difference: The Dictionary in the High School." *Counterpoints,* vol. 184, 2001, pp. 171–185. *JSTOR,* JSTOR, www.jstor.org/stable/42976661.

Resources

1. "Birth Control Methods." *Bedsider,* Power to Decide, www.bedsider.org /methods.

2. "Birth Control Methods." *Bedsider.*

3. "Birth Control Methods." *Bedsider.*

4. https://www.plannedparenthood.org/learn/birth-control/condom/how-effective -are-condoms.

5. "Birth Control Methods." *Bedsider.*

6. Rathus, Spencer A. et al. "Chapter 16: Sexually Transmitted Infections" In *Human Sexuality in a World of Diversity.* Pages 506–549. Seventh edition. Boston: Pearson, 2008.

7. Rathus, "Chapter 16 . . ." *Human Sexuality in a World of Diversity.*

8. Rathus, "Chapter 16 . . ." *Human Sexuality in a World of Diversity.*

9. Rathus, "Chapter 16 . . ." *Human Sexuality in a World of Diversity.*

10. Rathus, "Chapter 16 . . ." *Human Sexuality in a World of Diversity.*

11. Wald, Anna. "Investigational HPV Vaccine Shows 100% Efficacy." *NEJM Journal Watch,* 22 Nov. 2005, www.jwatch.org/wh200511220000001/2005/11/22 /investigational-hpv-vaccine-shows-100-efficacy.

12. "HPV and Men: CDC Fact Sheet." *Centers for Disease Control and Prevention,* 14 July 2017, www.cdc.gov/std/hpv/stdfact-hpv-and-men.htm.

13. Rathus, "Chapter 16 . . ." *Human Sexuality in a World of Diversity*

14. Singh, Neeta. "HPV and Cervical Cancer." *Cancer Research,* American Association for Cancer Research, 1 May 2008, cancerres.aacrjournals.org/content/68/9 _Supplement/4717.short.

15. "HPV and Men: CDC Fact Sheet." *Centers for Disease Control and Prevention*, 14 July 2017, www.cdc.gov/std/hpv/stdfact-hpv-and-men.htm.

16. Wald, Anna. "Investigational HPV Vaccine Shows 100% Efficacy." *NEJM Journal Watch,* 22 Nov. 2005, www.jwatch.org/wh200511220000001/2005/11/22/investigational-hpv-vaccine-shows-100-efficacy.

17. Wald, Anna. "Investigational HPV Vaccine Shows 100% Efficacy." *NEJM Journal Watch,* 22 Nov. 2005, www.jwatch.org/wh200511220000001/2005/11/22/investigational-hpv-vaccine-shows-100-efficacy.

18. Rathus, "Chapter 16 . . ." *Human Sexuality in a World of Diversity.*

19. Rathus, "Chapter 16 . . ." *Human Sexuality in a World of Diversity.*

20. "Hepatitis C Questions and Answers for the Public." *Centers for Disease Control and Prevention*, 12 June 2018, www.cdc.gov/hepatitis/hcv/cfaq.htm.

21. Rathus, "Chapter 16 . . ." *Human Sexuality in a World of Diversity.*

22. Rathus, "Chapter 16 . . ." *Human Sexuality in a World of Diversity.*

23. Rathus, "Chapter 16 . . ." *Human Sexuality in a World of Diversity.*

24. Rathus, "Chapter 16 . . ." *Human Sexuality in a World of Diversity.*

25. Rathus, "Chapter 16 . . ." *Human Sexuality in a World of Diversity.*

26. Rathus, "Chapter 16 . . ." *Human Sexuality in a World of Diversity.*

27. Rathus, "Chapter 16 . . ." *Human Sexuality in a World of Diversity.*

28. Rathus, "Chapter 16 . . ." *Human Sexuality in a World of Diversity.*

29. Rathus, "Chapter 16 . . ." *Human Sexuality in a World of Diversity.*

30. Rathus, "Chapter 16 . . ." *Human Sexuality in a World of Diversity.*

31. Rathus, "Chapter 16 . . ." *Human Sexuality in a World of Diversity.*

32. Rathus, "Chapter 16 . . ." *Human Sexuality in a World of Diversity.*

33. Rathus, "Chapter 16 . . ." *Human Sexuality in a World of Diversity.*

34. Rathus, "Chapter 16 . . ." *Human Sexuality in a World of Diversity.*

35. Rathus, "Chapter 16 . . ." *Human Sexuality in a World of Diversity.*

36. Rathus, "Chapter 16 . . ." *Human Sexuality in a World of Diversity.*

37. "Male Breast Cancer." *MedlinePlus*, U.S. National Library of Medicine, 23 Aug. 2018, medlineplus.gov/malebreastcancer.html.

38. Punukollu, M. "Self Breast Exam." *Women's Health Information*, Feminist Women's Health Center, 2011, www.fwhc.org/health/self-breast-exam.htm.

39.   Punukollu, M. "Self Breast Exam." *Women's Health Information*, Feminist
      Women's Health Center, 2011, www.fwhc.org/health/self-breast-exam.htm.

40.   Steamship Mutual. Sea Venture Vol. 18, June 1999. Accessed on 22 Aug. 2017,
      https://www.steamshipmutual.com/publications/Articles/Articles/Safe
      _Port.asp.

ACKNOWLEDGMENTS

Thank you to Tony Lyons of Skyhorse Publishing for your vision and for your willingness to take risks. To my editor, Caroline Russomanno, thank you for your care and consideration. You made this work even better. And thank you to my dedicated agent, Maryann Karinch of The Rudy Agency: our common goals and shared passions are changing the world, one word at a time.

A huge, resounding Thank You to my friends, my family, and my intentional community. Without you, this book (and I) certainly would not be here. Thank you for telling me the truth and for always leading by example. Thank you for your gentle nudges and for all of the attention, care, and love along the way. And also, for the many, many cups of tea.

Speaking of tea, thank you, Autumn Austin (fellow tea devotee), for your beautiful and thoughtful illustrations. Your astute eye has impressed me over and over. I appreciate your steadfast enthusiasm for this project and the message it represents, it was a true pleasure to work with you.

Mara Altman, thank you for your guidance and mentorship during this superb publishing journey. Your words of experience and encouragement have been invaluable, and I am grateful for our growing friendship.

Thank you, Daisy, for facilitating the initial draft of this text all those years ago and for your continual encouragement since then.

Amalia, I am immensely grateful for your enthusiastic contributions to this project. Thank you, in particular, for your resourcefulness.

Kim, thank you for not only teaching me how to read and write (thus providing me the essential tools for this task) but for being such a big voice of encouragement to *finish* this thing. We can now, officially, check this one off the list.

Thank you to my parents, of whom I refer to continuously throughout this text and throughout my life. Your will to live life as free human beings inspires me continually. Thank you for having the guts to raise me the best way you know how.

To my siblings, whom I am also proud to count as friends: you are brilliant joys in my life. This is for us.

And finally (as is fitting with your personal preference): thank you, Celine. Friend, teacher, confidant, you fill many roles in my life and without you, *On Blossoming* would still be but a bud. Thank you.

ABOUT THE AUTHOR

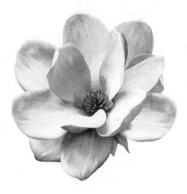

GIA LYNNE is a pleasure-positive writer, educator, and personal coach who is dedicated to researching and teaching the craft of pleasurable living and healthy sexuality. Fascinated by human sexuality and how that connects to our quality of life, she offers a unique perspective on pleasurable living. She has degree in English Literature from UC Berkeley and is pursuing a master's degree in Sexuality Studies.